THE FIRST DIET

TRANSFORM YOUR HEALTH WITH THE FOOD THAT MADE YOU HUMAN

BY: SEAN BISSELL

www.TheFirstDiet.com

TABLE OF CONTENTS

DISCLAIMER

The information included in this book is for educational and informational purposes only and is not intended as a substitute for the medical advice of a licensed physician. I am not a medical doctor, and any advice I give is my opinion based on my own experience. As such, you should always seek the advice of your own health care professionals before acting upon anything I publish or recommend. By reading this book you agree that my company and I are not responsible for your health or the health of your dependents. Any statements or claims about the possible health benefits conferred by any foods have not been evaluated by the Food and Drug Administration and are therefore not intended to diagnose, treat, cure, or prevent any disease.

ACKNOWLEDGEMENTS

I would like to thank my wife Lindsey for the time I took away from her and our family to write this book. Lindsey, your support and patience through this process is appreciated more than I could ever fully express here. I love you Lindsey, you are an astoundingly incredible wife, mother and friend.

Thank you to my parents for their unending support, help, guidance, love, and for always lending me their ears when I need help working through something.

And I would also like to thank my friend Karen McCormick for her inspiration and encouragement. Our chats were invaluable to the creation of this book. "Be as smart as you can, but know there's always more."
–Karen McCormick

A SPECIAL INVITATION

As the creator of The First Diet I felt it was my responsibility to create an online community where readers could go to connect, get encouragement, share ideas, and support one another. A place where they could discuss the book, post videos, and maybe swap some recipes, or exercise routines, and possibly find a friend or two.

Plus, as my way of saying thanks, if you join the group, you'll also get a free bonus audio chapter that's not available anywhere else.

To join the community, simply visit:
www.TheFirstDiet.com/community

Chapter 1

IMPORTANT: READ THIS BEFORE YOU BEGIN

Thank you for making the decision to read this book. I really appreciate you taking the time out of your life to understand the ideas behind The First Diet. As a new dad, I completely understand how valuable time is, and I know that reading a book takes a lot of time.

I did my best to make this book as short as possible while still explaining everything you need to know. Of course there will be questions no matter how thorough a book is, but I did my best to cover the critical points without overwhelming you. My goal was to give you enough information to understand and incorporate these ideas into your life. That is, if you would like to.

I feel a pressure to get right to the point, to tell you exactly what The First Diet is, what foods are included, and how to put all the pieces together. But I know if I did that, I would be doing you a massive disservice. I would be killing your ability to understand and use the ideas in The First Diet, because ideas without understanding are at best useless, and at worst dangerous.

Why do I know that if I cut to the chase I would be doing you harm? The modern world is in the middle of a massive health crisis. Obesity and Diabetes type 2 are at record levels[1,2]. Degenerative diseases and metabolic disorders are on the rise, and we need to turn this trend around[3].

I fully believe that The First Diet can help do this, and because of that, I need you to understand the ideas in this book. Unfortunately, if I told you these ideas right now, you wouldn't believe me.

Why won't you believe me? For the same reasons I didn't even believe myself in the beginning. I resisted these ideas. I didn't want to believe what I was discovering, and I didn't want to change what I was doing. Eventually, the evidence was too great, and my personal results convinced me. This is real, and this works.

But if you're like me, you need evidence. You need incredible reasons as to why something works. And you should need evidence to believe something. Believing everything you hear with no critical thought is the definition of gullible. If you're reading this book, I highly doubt you're gullible.

To protect ourselves from being gullible, and to protect against too many bad ideas competing in our brains, we have developed idea immune systems. These idea immune systems are primarily designed to protect us from harmful ideas, and for the most part this system works well. We don't believe everything we hear, and we kick out ideas that don't fit in with what we believe. Mostly this works to our benefit, but sometimes our idea immune system can get hijacked by negative sources.

It's difficult to notice when our idea immune system has been taken hostage, but it's happening more than ever today. The media have become true experts at influencing our idea immune systems. Specifically, the media uses sensational headlines and stories spun in a way to instill a unique combination of trust and fear. This combination secretly whispers into our ears, "Trust me, I'm important, this is true." They often do this by piggy-backing on an expert's opinion—taken out of context—or by twisting a study's conclusions to make a shocking headline.

The media needs a villain to get people to listen. And as the saying goes, "If it bleeds, it leads." Fear can reliably bypass our idea immune systems and trick us to be gullible. For example, if you suddenly heard a voice screaming, "Look out! Duck!" you would probably look around and start to duck. There would be no critical thought or analysis of the source of the information. Instantly your belief changed from, "I am safe," to, "I'm in danger!" Fear is powerful, and if the media is able to scare us into believing something is bad for us, then as long as we are scared, our idea immune system will reject any effort to believe new information coming in that says otherwise.

The media is constantly shouting, "Look out! Duck!" It's difficult to resist the corruption of our idea immune system by the media. No one is completely immune, so please do not feel bad if you have fallen victim to this exploitation. I know I've been fooled many times before. It's hard to tell when your idea immune system has been hijacked and is causing you to be wrong about something. Because the feeling of being right and the feeling of being wrong is exactly the same, until the moment you realize you were wrong.

I am fully aware I am going to be fighting many idea immune systems in this book. Mine put up a struggle when I was discovering the foundation of The First Diet. It's because of this idea battle that I must present the information in this book in a deliberate way that starts even before the beginning.

Please bear with me as I unravel this web, even if you don't learn the full details of The First Diet until later in this book. The way this information is laid out is important for your understanding. I want you to have fun and discover new things, even before the full details of The First Diet are revealed.

Chapter 2

WHAT THIS BOOK WILL SHOW YOU

The first human remains were found in Ethiopia, dated at 200,000 years ago[1,2]. During that time, Ethiopia was a warm and tropical climate[3,4]. It is likely that we evolved to be humans in this hot environment.

And you're hot, too. The human body is 98.6 degrees on average[5]. You probably know what it feels like to be in 98.6 degree weather. It's warm, and you're a warm blooded human. Each human is made of approximately 37 trillion cells, all bathing in the tropical 98.6 degree weather of your warm blooded body[6].

But recently we've forgotten our tropical past. We've been tricked into eating mostly cold-weather foods. We've been eating like coldblooded beings, and we are paying a price for it.

Scientists can see what people have been eating by examining their cells. Studies show that in the year 1960[7], eight percent of people's fat tissues in the U.S. were made of "cold weather" fat. In 2008 that number jumped to twenty-five percent[8].

Now contrast that with the fact that in the year 1960, thirteen percent of people in the U.S. were obese. In 2010 that number increased to thirty-five percent[9]. That's a 310% increase in "cold weather" fat in our tissues and a 270% increase in obesity—a close tie in numbers.

In addition, the total caloric sweeteners eaten in the U.S. took a sharp decline around 1998, which did nothing to stop the obesity epidemic. From 1998 to 2010, sugar consumption dropped by 15%[10], and while people in the U.S. were eating less sugar, the number of obese individuals went up by approximately 37%[11,9].

Why is this happening? Why are people sicker today more than ever before? This is largely a result of damaged metabolisms due to metabolic-fuel-incompatibility. Giving your warm-blooded body cold-weather foods is like putting diesel fuel in a gasoline car: Guaranteed to give bad results.

This damage can be reversed; the human body is resilient. In order to heal, we must eat foods proven to stabilize and increase metabolic function, the foods that grew where we evolved and became human. The same foods that gave us so much metabolic energy we could afford to evolve such a large brain. But as we'll explore later, even our brain size is in jeopardy if we do not change the way we eat, and soon.

The First Diet is focused on showing you the foods compatible with our 98.6 degree bodies, create more energy and help increase your metabolism. This is the same type of energy that helped us evolve into the big-brained humans we are today.

This book may also erase some long standing fears of foods you may have. The media does a good job of trying to scare people away from some of the healthiest foods you could possibly eat. The First Diet will help untangle the damage the media has done and free up many new healthy and tasty food choices to you.

In this book, you will discover the science behind a new and more fun way to eat, a way that will open new food possibilities for those who have been influenced by the media's scare tactics. With the knowledge contained in this book, you can be a "health nut in disguise." You can be healthy, possibly even lose weight, and no one would even know you're following a diet because you won't be avoiding "unhealthy" foods. You won't look like you're trying to eat healthy at all. People might just think you have a secret, or that you just have great genetics. But you'll know the truth.

In The First Diet, you will discover, in detail, how your body uses food for energy. Understanding how this really works can help you optimize your metabolism and avoid falling for bad diet information in the future. After reading The First Diet, you will be able to stand your ground and feel confident in what you know. You'll be able to tell when someone is just trying to scare you into watching something, buying something, or influencing your behavior. Reading this book will help you gain solid ground and confidence over your diet choices.

The First Diet will show you combinations of foods that will help you increase your metabolism naturally and healthily. Boosting your metabolic rate is imperative because a healthy metabolism almost always leads to greater health and longevity. But it is important to know that trying to create a healthy metabolism does not always lead to weight loss. Rather, it often does the exact opposite. Understanding the difference between a healthy metabolism and weight loss is extremely important. This book will show you ways to keep a healthy metabolism while losing weight.

Additionally, The First Diet will help you understand how you can retain or gain muscle and become stronger. You will learn ways to keep or increase your muscle mass and strength without expensive supplements or fancy workout routines.

Chapter 3

MY STORY

Nutrition and diet are two of the most confusing topics anyone could ever discuss. The human body is one of the most complex "machines" you could conceivably study. Understanding what makes us work and how to use that to our advantage can seem like a never-ending undertaking.

What makes things even more confusing is that our bodies are able to survive on many different types of diets. Humans can eat a surprising variety of foods and not only survive, but thrive. Some live into old age eating many different types of foods and with strikingly different lifestyles, all over the world.

This ability of our bodies to use many different foods, and live long happy lives, makes finding the "optimal" diet extremely challenging. While technically you can live in the Arctic and eat seal fat and fish all day long, is that the best thing for your body? Could you potentially feel better and live longer while eating something different?

Lifestyle, genetics, family, your upbringing, culture, your social hierarchy, and many other factors come into play in determining how you feel, how your body performs, and how long you live. Nutrition has a place, but you cannot completely isolate nutrition from your life. You have to live your life around food; the two cannot be detached. Because of this, separating out diet, genetics, culture, happiness, etc. is almost completely impossible, and will most likely never be achieved.

Focusing on isolated and specific factors surrounding nutrition has also led many nutritionists to false conclusions that look good on paper, but end up leading people away from optimal health instead of toward it. To make matters worse, identifying how your body reacts to certain foods and quantities is complicated enough on its own. As a result of this confusion, nutrition often becomes nothing more than a guessing game based in myths, traditions, and stories.

History, traditions, and our fossil records can reveal enlightening stories about our nutritional roots, but we must be careful to cross reference the stories we tell with scientific truth, and we must keep in mind that just because we may have eaten a specific way in the past, that does not necessarily mean it is the optimal diet now.

In order to come up with an ideal diet for humans, we must look into the past, and find out what made us human. We must discover what diet we thrived on in our early years. We need to overlay that information on our modern bodies, and our modern times. We must find clues from the past, and modify them for our current environment and biology, and this must all be done in a way that uses the science of nutrition as a guide and a cross reference.

For example, if anthropology tells us we ate a specific plant in the past, and now nutritional science tells us that plant is poisonous, then we should not incorporate that plant into our modern times.

That is exactly what this book is going to do. The First Diet will look back into human's history and explore key aspects of our nutritional past. We will discover what made us thrive, cross reference that with science, and then suggest ways to modify it for our modern world.

But first, who am I and why should you trust me anyway? Well, let me tell you my story.

Growing up, I was never into nutrition. I didn't really care what I ate, as long as it tasted good. My parents, on the other hand, did care—my mom specifically.

She never talked to us about why she thought something was "healthy" or not. However, she did try to cook us healthy meals. To her, that meant whole grains instead of refined grains, and not a great deal of sweets. We ate a variety of vegetables, fruits, meat, fish, eggs, etc., and no fast food. She always made us a bagged lunch for school instead of eating the cafeteria food. My mom tried to make things taste as good as possible. She was, and still is, a great cook.

My dad routinely told my brother and I, "Your mom is looking out for us in the kitchen." We left it up to her that our nutrition would work out for the best. Looking back on things, I think my mom really was onto something even though she never did any formal research into the subject of nutrition.

My mom's cooking was a blessing, and also in a small part a curse. She was cooking on a "hunch" and could never truly articulate why she was doing what she was doing. That meant I could never really replicate what she did, except for copying exactly what she did, which did not allow for self-reliance or creativity in the area of nutrition. Additionally, having all of my meal planning and cooking done for me caused me to essentially forget about nutrition altogether. I never needed to think about it, so I never explored the topic for myself.

When I eventually went off to college on my own, and no longer was under the wing of my mom's nutrition, I ate cafeteria food pretty much exclusively for a year. Then after that year I joined a fraternity where we had a heroin addicted cook who did anything she could to make cooking easier on herself. That naturally gravitated to deep fat frying everything possible. I even saw a deep fat fried apple.

We had huge 5 gallon tubs of partially hydrogenated soybean oil that would stay in the fryer until it was tar black from not getting changed frequently enough. Eventually we'd get rid of the black-tar and refill the 5 gallons of soy oil into our two industrial fryers and start over.

Beyond the deep fat fryer grease-filled food, we always had two 5 gallon tubs of sugary, cheap artificially flavored, Kool-Aid knockoff drinks that we'd mix up daily and have sitting on the counter so we could drink it throughout the day.

Pretty much all the food was frozen in bags ready to deep fry, or there was an artificial cheese substance ready to make grilled cheese sandwiches drenched in margarine. Or some other type of fake fat, chemically flavored, food-like-substance. My diet looked like this for about three straight years—including the cafeteria food, which was better than the fraternity food, but not by much.

During my time in the fraternity, there were some older members who were into lifting weights and were "huge" from my perspective, as a 135 pound scrawny kid. They took me under their wing and showed me how to lift weights in a bodybuilder's fashion. I started lifting more, eating more of the heroin addict's food preparations, and got great results. I bulked up from 135 pounds to 185 at my highest. I felt strong, and was proud of my gains.

Although I was proud of my newfound muscle, I was starting to feel bad in the gym. After heavy deadlifts, I would start to get dizzy and nauseated. Taking a powerful multivitamin aimed at bodybuilders seemed to help offset that a bit. Looking back on things, I should have realized I was having significant nutritional deficiencies through my fraternity diet.

I also started to supplement with meal replacement shakes, which had some vitamins and minerals in them as well. But almost everything I was eating was artificial in some way, whether artificial flavorings, artificially created foods, or lab-created vitamins.

Eventually, I got to the point where if I did a heavy squat session, I would end up on the floor writhing in pain from the worst headaches I've ever had. They were so bad I was completely immobilized, and couldn't even stand up. And there was nothing I could do but wait out the pain on the floor.

At that time I was in the "power thorough it, no pain no gain" mentality, so it took a few of those horrible headaches to realize something bad was happening. One particularly horrible headache that felt ten times worse than a strong brain freeze, combined with cold sweats and extreme nausea, motivated me to go see a doctor. The doctor referred me to a specialist, and I ended up in the hospital getting a CAT scan.

After the CAT scan, the doctor showed me the pictures of my head, and pointed to a troubling plaque buildup in the arteries of my neck going up to my brain. The specialist was visibly disturbed by this and told me this type of buildup is serious and should not happen at my age. And no matter what age, it was a bad situation to be in.

Unfortunately, they didn't offer me any solutions, and they didn't ask anything about my diet. I was in so much shock at the time, I hardly remember anything past that point in the visit.

That picture of my arteries shook me up so much that after the shock wore off, I started on a massive research binge. I needed to know what could be causing this issue, and what I could do to stop it from progressing or to reverse it.

My research led me to trans fats, made from vegetable oil. And it was easy to see that my diet had been abnormally high in cold-weather fats. This was mostly due to the large amounts of partially hydrogenated soy oil from the deep fat fryer grease—but margarine and many other fraternity foods also played a part.

I immediately stopped eating the foods provided to us from the kitchen, and started making my own meals based on my newfound knowledge. I also cut out trans fats as much as humanly possible. It took some time, but eventually the headaches stopped. I slowly started to feel better than I had in years, and my improvement showed me that nutrition can have a huge impact on your health, energy levels, how you look, and your athletic performance.

Because of these obvious improvements in my health, I started researching nutrition more and more. At first, this research was born out of necessity, and eventually it became something I genuinely found fun.

Since that time, I have looked into many diets. I've personally tested out at least 10 variations over the years. I tried many out of curiosity, and some were an attempt to reach specific goals. Some worked well, while others created more problems than they fixed. I have more embarrassing stories about diet failures than I care to admit.

When I tried a diet variation, I would become interested in the practical application, but I would also dive into the mechanics and theory as much as I could. I wanted to figure out what was going on behind the scenes and understand what the diet was supposed to be doing on a scientific level.

Results that come from a diet are equally, if not more important, than the practical application and theory. I also learned that results are often deceiving and therefore must be taken with skepticism. For example, a popular weight loss diet may help people lose weight quickly, but that same diet could end up causing health problems three years later. Or maybe someone feels instantly energetic on a new diet, but after a year into their plan, they crash from exhaustion.

When something burns out, it starts off bright, strong, and vibrant—until the fire burns out and there's only a smoldering heap of ash left. Because of this phenomenon, long term results are almost always more important than short term. Sometimes it's better to shine less bright in the beginning so you don't completely burn out later. When starting any new diet or modification, long term results should be one of the first considerations.

I know this because I've tried a ton of diets in my exploration, from low-carb, to low-fat, to low-protein, to high-carb, to high-fat, to high-protein; from ancestral-diets, to low-calorie-high-nutrient-diets, to high-calorie-low-nutrient-diets; from gluten-free, to carb-free, to grains-free, to sugar-free; from whole foods, to processed foods, to "just eat real food," to "if it fits your macros"; from no-supplements to tons-of-supplements, to weird-unheard-of-supplements, and beyond. If there's a diet out there, I've probably tried it or at least researched it.

Through all the diet variations I've tested, and all the research—all the conversations I've had over 14 years—I now have a deeper understanding of nutrition than I ever aspired to achieve. Throughout my research, I stumbled upon something hidden in plain sight that I believe takes a holistic and comprehensive view of our evolutionary history, combined with science, physiology, biology, and psychology—and it is evidence-based and results-driven. What I have found has helped myself, my family, and many others I know. I want to share it with you.

I owe my discovery to many people whose work and research I drew my findings from. Without the effort of many others, I would never have come to the conclusions I have today. I appreciate them greatly. There are countless unnamed researchers who have discovered and explained how our bodies' metabolic processes work, how our psychology influences our biology, and how exercise can influence both. Some mentionables include, Sir Hans Adolf Krebs, Ray Peat, Howard Bloom, Hans Selye, Mark Sisson, Loren Cordain, Carol Dweck, and Daniel Kaheneman. Although I don't agree with all the people I have named, I am grateful because without them, I wouldn't know what I do agree with. Lastly, I'd like to thank those who have led me astray, because without my failures, I would not appreciate what I know now.

Maybe I should have put more thank yous at the beginning of this book, but I list them now to illustrate that I did not come up with these ideas on my own, and this book is a synthesis of many smart people's work and ideas. It took me many years to finally see how all these ideas and theories fit together, and how strangely simple and obvious the answer is that I've arrived at.

However, all of the pieces of this revelation didn't come together easily for me. In fact, in the beginning I resisted the information. I tried to disprove it because it went against almost everything I knew. But I was lucky enough that my research gave me a strong background in nutrition, and despite my resistance, I was able to see the truth, and let the truth change my outlook on nutrition. If I was less experienced, I may have created a fictitious story to explain away the facts, to preserve my view on nutrition and make myself feel mentally better. Today, I am grateful I worked through my previous bias and saw a bigger picture, and I want you to see that picture, too. If you understand and internalize the concepts this book will discuss, you will inevitably change your life.

I call what I found "The First Diet" and I believe what is in The First Diet is vital to the health of humanity, especially in today's modern society where diseases like obesity and Diabetes type 2 are running rampant. The First Diet has the potential to give humanity a fresh start, more energy, less disease, improved moods, easier going kids, less worry about diet. In short, it provides healthier and happier people. That's the goal of The First Diet, to make people all over the world healthier and happier.

Chapter 4

HOW THE CAVEMAN DIET TOOK A CHUNK OUT OF MY BRAIN THE SIZE OF A TENNIS BALL

Perhaps the most important trait humans developed over time is our exceptionally large brains. Along with monkeys and apes, humans are technically primates, and brain size is a key factor in determining a primate's intelligence[32]. Compared to other animals, the average primate brain is 1.9 times bigger than it would be expected to be based on the size of their bodies, and primates have significant intelligence[33]. But that doesn't even come close to the human brain capacity. For contrast, human's brains are 7 times larger than they should be for their body size[34]. The large brain and intelligence of humans is likely the reason why the Latin word for humans is Homo sapiens; because translated, Homo sapiens means "wise person."

Humans first evolved in tropical and tropical-savanna Africa[1]. It was an environment with many food resources, like meat from animals, tubers, leafy greens, and fruit[2,3,4].

Life is never easy, but in regards to food resources, evolving humans likely had it pretty good. That is, until the drought happened. It hit shortly after we evolved into who we are today, Homo sapiens[5]. And it appears to have hit so hard that the water receded enough where a land bridge opened and gave access to Europe, India and Asia[6].

Given the opportunity, those humans would have probably stayed in Africa. But with droughts come a lack of food and water. Animals died, tubers were hard to find, leafy greens disappeared, and fruit became scarce[7].

Our early human ancestors were forced to leave to find greener pastures. Some stayed to fight it out in the drought, but many left[8,9] and life became hard. Fruit and sugar were scarce. But other opportunities opened up, and you probably know what happened next if you are familiar with the Paleo diet.

Humans became "cavemen," building fires in the cold, hunting for food, gathering as much as they could[10,11], moving around from place to place like the nomads they were[12]. Food was scarce for many, but they made it work, and we hung on until agriculture was invented[13].

After agriculture, life changed for humans. We settled down, stopped being nomadic, and we domesticated animals[13,14]. Sugar was still limited for the most part and grains had dominated our carbohydrate sources[15], but at least there was food.

While life was better for most, and nutrition was more available, there is a secret about human evolution not often spoke of. Since we left Africa, our brains have been slowly shrinking. We have lost a chunk of brain mass the size of a tennis ball, from the time we were born as humans in Africa to our present day[16].

There is a great deal of speculation as to why that happened. Some think our brains are becoming more efficient and we don't need the extra space, while some think we are losing the parts of our brains that make us aggressive. Others believe we are becoming dumber, as living in cities is easier and we don't need as much brain power to operate in them[16]. I think there's another angle that hasn't been explored, and is somewhat controversial.

When we were forced to leave Africa, we also left our abundant sugar sources. We abandoned our fruit and palm trees. We ended up finding enough calories through other sources, but it was not ideal. Our brains are 2% of our body weight, and take up 20% of our energy[17]. Human brains may have even taken up more energy 200,000 years ago. Having a large brain is not exactly energy efficient. Our brains need carbohydrates to function[18], and carbohydrates promote a higher energy metabolism[19].

But if you are starving, having a large brain that takes up 20% or more of your energy is not a great idea. In the situation of a chronic energy shortage, evolution would try to bring our brain size down in order to compensate, and it seems to have done that[16]. Brains all over the world have shrunken, and the smallest reported human brains now belong to the Bushmen in Africa, and the Aboriginal people in Australia[20]. This does not include pygmy people in Africa, as their brains are the smallest, but so are their bodies, so we'll discuss them later[20].

What would cause the Bushmen and Aboriginal people to have the smallest brain sizes? If you look at their diet, there are clues. Bushmen have a high-fat low-carbohydrate diet, and sometimes a very low-carbohydrate diet[21]. Their staple food is the mongongo nut, which is mostly fat[22.]. As for their animal sources, they hunt by running their prey into exhaustion, known as persistence hunting[23]. Hunters can run after their prey for days with little food to eat, until their prey falls down from exhaustion and the hunter can kill it and bring it home. Because of the highly energy-intensive hunting, combined with the low carbohydrate diet, it is likely that the Bushmen have downregulated their brain size to take up less energy and to better survive[24].

The Aboriginal people in Australia have a low calorie, high nutrient dense diet[25]. The calories they get are in a form of feast and famine. There are many periods of famine and short burst of feasting[25]. They get little sugar, but when they come across honey or other sources, they devour it as a delicacy[25]. On average, though, the Aboriginal people rely on small amounts of calories, and therefore evolution has likely downregulated their brain size to take up less energy[24].

And what about the smallest brains and bodies of all human populations anywhere on Earth? Those belong to the pygmy tribes[20]. Historically, pygmy people have had a difficult time getting enough food on a consistent basis[26]. The lack of consistent food combined with disease has shortened pygmy people's life spans significantly. On average, the lifespan of a human pygmy is from 16-24 years of age[27]. Only 30-50% of children survive to 15 years of age[27]. And less than a third of women live to see menopause at 37[27].

It is because of this lack of nutrition, and lowered lifespan that the pygmy bodies were forced to start reproducing at younger and younger ages[27]. And younger people have smaller bodies. But this is counterintuitive, because generally people who grow taller and larger tend to be more fertile and birth larger and more robust offspring. That's obviously a good thing for survival, but not if the average lifespan is so low that adults may not have a chance to have children at all. In this hazardous situation, nature favours those who mature and reproduce early, at the cost of their growth.

The smallest recorded brains belong to the Bushmen, the Aboriginal people, and pygmies[20]. These populations get small amounts of carbohydrates, and little calories, at least compared to other more "neolithic" or "industrialized" parts of the world[21,25,26,27]. Now that's all interesting, but what pulls this all together is that recently anthropology has shown us that our brains have begun to grow once again. They stopped shrinking, and started growing right around the time of the American colonies[16]. What does this also line up with in history? The sugar trade[28].

That's right, at the same time that sugar once again became a staple in the human diet, our brains stopped shrinking and started expanding again[16]. Take away sugar, and brains start to shrink; bring back sugar, and brains start to grow.

Having a big brain is a luxury in the natural world. There are plenty of organisms that do just fine and live long lives without big brains. Before we became humans, we happened to be at the right place at the right time in the tropical environment of Africa[29]. That supplied us with energy-rich sugar sources and gave our biology signals of abundant brain energy[30].

Because there was an abundance of brain energy, Homo sapiens had an opportunity to let our brains grow, develop and get bigger. However, if you take away that brain energy, evolution must keep going, but it will adapt back down, and find ways to conserve—likely by shrinking our brains again[24]. In fact, brain shrinkage also happens to occur with Diabetes type 2. Diabetes type 2 is defined by the inability to use blood sugar correctly and studies now show that Diabetes type 2 can lead to significant brain volume reduction[31].

Chapter 5

WHY SUGAR IS GOOD FOR YOU

I don't know when you're reading this book, but at the time I'm writing it, sugar has a bad reputation. Sugar is under attack from a giant anti-sugar smear campaign. I have no idea what the motivation behind the attack on sugar is. It may be just a fad, it may be deliberately created by some evil genius, or it may be honest confusion. Whatever it is, people are afraid of sugar right now[1].

Sugar is being blamed for almost every disease under the sun from sugar lowering your immune system and causing you to catch the common cold, to sugar causing Diabetes type 2, and worse[2,3]. There are entire feature-length documentaries that paint sugar as an evil substance, and compare it to cocaine for its so-called addictive nature. I'm sure someone will say that I'm protecting sugar in this book because I'm addicted to it.

But none of that is true. It's mass hysteria and overhyped negativity. Sugar is not the evil substance it's made out to be. In fact, sugar is one of the most powerful substances we can include in our diet, and as the last chapter showed, sugar is likely responsible for keeping our brains healthy and potentially even increasing our intelligence.

Yes, you can overeat on sugar, and yes that can cause problems. But that is true with any type of food. You can overeat on fat, you can overeat on sugar, and you can overeat on protein. However, protein is challenging to eat too much of, and it's frankly disgusting for most people to eat 3,000 calories of protein.

And just like protein, it would be difficult to overeat on sugar. It would get sickening to eat 3,000 calories of pure sugar for most people, which is

187 teaspoons. Can you imagine eating that much sugar in a day, every day?

The truth of the matter is, sugar isn't addictive; really great tasting food is addictive—and easy to overeat[4]. Usually really great tasting food contains a combination of sugar, and fat. Think doughnuts, cookies, chocolate, etc. Even foods that don't have sugar, and instead have a combination of plain old carbohydrates and fat can be addictive. Think potato chips, French fries, pizza, etc. Great chefs have created addictive food[5]. Sugar on its own is not addictive; sugar is pretty gross in its purest form.

If people were truly addicted to sugar, they would be going for the pure stuff, and lots of it. Drug addicts don't want their drugs cut with filler; they want the purest, strongest drugs possible. If true sugar addicts exist, they would not want their sugar watered down in a soda, or mixed in with a cookie—they would be shoveling pure white sugar straight into their mouths. However, people don't eat sugar straight.

But doesn't sugar turn into fat? The short answer to that question is no[6]. The long answer is that the process of sugar turning into fat is called "de novo lipogenesis," which rarely happens in humans in any significant quantity. The truth is, the fat you eat is already fat, and is stored in your body as fat[7]. The sugar you eat is already sugar and is stored in your body as sugar. There is no magical insulin fairy that waves her magic insulin wand and turns sugar into fat.

But what about fructose? If you know about the so-called evils of fructose, then you are well aware of the smear campaign against sugar. But fructose is not the evil substance it's said to be. In fact, fructose is exactly what makes sugar such the powerful health promoting substance it can be. And you will see why in a moment. But first we need to cover some sugar basics.

Firstly, I need to say that I am not going to cite sources for every definition explained in this book, or for any claim that is under the umbrella of basic biochemistry. Medical studies do not cover basic biochemistry. Questions like, "How are carbohydrates metabolized?" or, "What are the different types of sugars?" are not easily answered in studies; they are answered in textbooks and encyclopedias. So if you want further reading on these subjects, please consult those sources[7,8,9,10].

Sugar can come from many different sources, and the term sugar is often used to describe more than one substance, especially in scientific papers. That can make the term "sugar" confusing. Just to make sure we're on the same page, let's go over a few different ways to use the word sugar. Then we'll decide on one definition to use for the rest of this book.

Scientifically speaking, sugar basically refers to a handful of carbohydrates. Some of the big classifications are monosaccharides, disaccharides, and oligosaccharides. Those sound complicated, but they're really just confusing words for simple ideas.

Monosaccharide basically means there's only one type of carbohydrate that is isolated, with "mono" meaning one. The most commonly referred to monosaccharide is glucose, like the glucose in your blood.

Disaccharide means that there are two different types of carbohydrates connected together, with "di" meaning two. The most commonly referred to disaccharide is table sugar, or "sucrose." Table sugar is made from two types of sugars stuck together. Those two sugars are glucose and fructose. When those two sugars are connected, like in table sugar, they make a "disaccharide."

Oligosaccharide means there are "a few" carbohydrates connected together, with the "oligo" meaning few. Sometimes you will hear oligosaccharides referred to as "polysaccharides," which also basically mean "many carbohydrates." Oligosaccharides are mostly found in plants, like vegetables, grains and potatoes. These are often referred to as starches.

So, technically speaking, potatoes, rice, wheat, asparagus, kale, and table sugar are all sugar. They're either a monosaccharide sugar, a disaccharide sugar, or an oligosaccharide sugar.

This gets confusing because when you're speaking to your friends you probably only really refer to "sugar" as the sugar you find in refined table sugar, the sugar found in sodas, or the sugar you add to cookies. But then a news report comes out and says that when you eat potatoes your body converts that potato right into sugar. While that is a true statement, they're twisting terminology to "shock" the general public. Because, while it's scientifically accurate to say potatoes turn into sugar in your blood, what they really mean is that potatoes turn into glucose in your blood, and glucose is a type of sugar. But glucose is not table sugar.

Blood sugar is also called "blood glucose." Blood glucose is a less confusing and more accurate statement than saying "blood sugar." It's more descriptive to say blood glucose instead of blood sugar.

Really boiling this down to its simplest level, most "sugar" you find in the grocery stores will exclusively end up as glucose in your bloodstream. The only exception to this rule is sucrose, which is the primary ingredient in table sugar, fruit, or honey.

Going forward in this book, when we say "sugar," we're going to be talking about sucrose, which is half glucose and half fructose. And when we were talking about sugar increasing brain size earlier in the book, it was also the same sugar we're talking about here. This is the same stuff found in fruit, honey, and white refined sugar, the sweet type of sugar.

So when people say "sugar" is bad, unless they're referring to carbohydrates in general, then they're most likely really saying, "Fructose is bad." Because when we're talking about carbohydrates, the only practical thing separating white sugar, fruit, or honey from a potato is fructose.

But is fructose really all that bad? To understand the answer to that question we first need to focus on the details of how carbohydrates are used for energy in your body.

Carbohydrates contain six carbons in their structure. In order for carbohydrates to be fully broken down and used for their maximum energy potential, all six of those carbons have to be broken apart from each other.

Every time they break apart, energy is created that your body can use later. When all six carbons are broken away from each other, you are then left with six molecules of carbon dioxide, which you breathe out through your lungs. This quantity of carbon dioxide is important, and you will see why later. But for now, just remember carbohydrates have six carbon molecules, and can release six carbon dioxide molecules.

There are three major parts to how your body breaks down the six carbons in carbohydrates and uses them for energy once they've gotten into your cells.

Part one is glycolysis.

Glycolysis is the process of breaking glucose in half. This creates two sugars called "pyruvate sugars", which are three carbons each. When fructose is broken in half, the process is called fructolysis, which also gives you two "pyruvate sugars." So at this point, glucose and fructose are identical, because they both make the exact same pyruvate sugars.

Both glycolysis and fructolysis don't need oxygen to work, and the process of them breaking in half and creating pyruvate sugars is done inside your cell, but outside of your mitochondria. Mitochondria are the "power plants" of your cells and they are like little cells inside your cells. They create most of energy your body runs on. But in the first step of carbohydrate metabolism, your mitochondria are not involved, and neither is oxygen.

Did you catch that? I'll repeat it because it's important. Once fructose or glucose gets into your cell and starts to be broken down for energy—past this first step of glycolysis or fructolysis—fructose and glucose are identical. They both are turned into the exact same substance called "pyruvate sugars." Past this point it doesn't matter if you ate a potato or straight refined white sugar, so the difference between table sugar and a potato must really be before this step—before the fructose or glucose even gets into your cells.

You'll see this difference shortly, but first, we need to go through the full carbohydrate metabolic process. This is important to see so you can understand where things can go right and wrong with carbohydrate metabolism.

Carbohydrate metabolism should be able to go beyond just turning carbohydrates into pyruvate. Because if you only get to the step of pyruvate, only a small amount of energy has been made for your body to use. It only snapped the 6 chain of carbon in half and stopped. It should be able to break all 6 of those bonds, not just one. But if you understand that carbohydrate metabolism can end here, then you can begin to see why some people have issues with carbohydrates.

Without enough oxygen, pyruvate sugars can't get used by your mitochondria. So if you are out of breath, or if you are exercising in a way that requires more oxygen than you have available, the pyruvate sugars won't get used by your mitochondria. That means the pyruvate sugars won't have anywhere to go inside your cell, they won't be broken down and they can start to pile up. In other words, if you ate any carbohydrates, a potato, or sugar, and if you don't have enough oxygen available, then those carbohydrates can get inside your cell, turned into pyruvate, and then do nothing. The process stops at pyruvate if there is not enough oxygen. So then what happens?

If pyruvate sugars sit unused for very long at all, they will turn into lactic acid. This is why, if you're exercising, or don't have enough oxygen in your system, you can start to build up lactic acid. Lactic acid can exit your cell and go back into your bloodstream. Your liver can turn lactic acid right back into glucose, which then can be used by your cells later. So if you could turn glucose into pyruvate, but you didn't have enough oxygen for your mitochondria to use that pyruvate, then pyruvate can turn into lactic acid, and then back to glucose. Once lactic acid turns back into glucose, your body can transform the glucose into pyruvate again, and try again to get it into your mitochondria.

If your mitochondria never get enough oxygen, or if your mitochondria are damaged in some way, then carbohydrate metabolism may stop here. If it does stop here at pyruvate, then carbohydrates will constantly recycle between glucose, to pyruvate to lactic acid, back to glucose, and the cycle repeats. In this case carbohydrates are not able to be used by your mitochondria—this can happen in Diabetes type 2. However, in most everyone, their mitochondria will be able to use the pyruvate sugars, and the process of breaking down pyruvate sugars is done in the Krebs Cycle.

This first step is important, so let's recap. Why can carbohydrate metabolism end here, by just making pyruvate and stopping? It stops here because pyruvate is unable to get into your mitochondria because of two primary reasons: because there is not enough oxygen for your mitochondria to use the pyruvate, or your mitochondria is damaged and cannot use the pyruvate, even if there is enough oxygen.

But you really want to be able to get past this stage and have the pyruvate get used by your mitochondria, which produces the most energy for your body, so you want your carbohydrates to get in there, and get turned into energy.

Next you will see what happens if your carbohydrates can be used by your mitochondria and what your mitochondria does with carbohydrates.

Part two is the Krebs Cycle.

Once you have pyruvate sugars, which are three carbons long each, they need to be broken apart even further by your mitochondria. This "breaking apart" happens inside the Krebs Cycle. For the Krebs Cycle to start, you need the pyruvate sugars to get inside your mitochondria and react with oxygen. If pyruvate can get into your mitochondria, and there is oxygen available, your mitochondria will then split apart all of the carbons that held the carbohydrates together. That will leave you with six carbon dioxide molecules, which you will breathe out through your lungs. After the carbohydrates are broken apart completely, you will have some "bite sized food" for your mitochondria to turn into raw energy. This energy creation is done in the electron transport chain.

Part three is the Electron Transport Chain.

Once the six carbon chain is broken in half by glycolysis or fructolysis, and the Krebs Cycle breaks down the rest, then the energy they created by splitting the carbons apart is ready to be used to create molecules called ATP. ATP is like pure energy for your body to live on, and the most ATP is made by your mitochondria in the Electron Transport Chain.

This is a complicated process, but here's a simplified explanation. The "bite sized food" energy created by splitting the pyruvate sugars apart runs in and out along the inner and outer membrane of your mitochondria. That builds enough momentum to eventually push together an ATP molecule. This energy momentum is kind of like shooting an energetic "ray gun" at a molecule called ADP, and that "ray gun" transforms ADP into ATP.

The carbohydrates created the energy for the "ray gun" of your mitochondria to fire at ADP and create ATP, and ATP is the fuel your body uses to live on. So it's not really the carbohydrates that your body runs on, it's actually the ATP.

Now that we understand how carbohydrates are used for energy in our bodies, it is important to understand that fats are also metabolized in similar ways. Once fats hit "step two," the Kreb's Cycle, then everything is almost identical between fat and carbohydrates being used for energy. They both do the same things in the Kreb's Cycle and the Electron Transport Chain. They both create ATP.

Fats, however, do not go through the "first step," glycolysis or fructolysis, It is in large part because fats don't use glycolysis or fructolysis that they produce less carbon dioxide than carbohydrates. Carbon dioxide is often classified as a "waste" product of your metabolism because you breathe it out like "exhaust" from a car. That is true on some level, because too much carbon dioxide can be poisonous, but too much oxygen can be equally poisonous.

The truth of the matter is that, just like oxygen, you need carbon dioxide to survive. Carbon dioxide helps red blood cells deliver oxygen to your cells. This phenomenon is referred to as the "Bohr effect." The Bohr effect basically says that an increase in carbon dioxide helps red blood cells release oxygen into cells, and a decrease in carbon dioxide makes red blood cells hold onto oxygen more. Simply stated, if you have too little carbon dioxide, then even if you have enough oxygen in your blood, your cells won't be able to use the oxygen.

There needs to be an optimal balance of carbon dioxide and oxygen for your body to work well. And having a normal carbohydrate metabolism helps bump up your carbon dioxide levels to more favorable ranges. In fact, there is some evidence that suggests living at a higher elevation that has less oxygen and more carbon dioxide can lower your cancer risk.

Optimal carbon dioxide levels help you use oxygen better. And remember, your mitochondria need oxygen to be able to go through the Kreb's Cycle and the Electron Transport Chain. Without enough oxygen, those processes can slow down. And those processes slowing down means your metabolism is slowing down.

So now that we understand a big part of why carbohydrate metabolism is important, why is fructose specifically important? Let's first start with why many people, especially the media, believe that fructose is bad for your health. And then we will look at those claims in more detail.

Here are the major reasons fructose is said to be a harmful substance.

- The majority of fructose goes straight to your liver, like other toxic substances, such as alcohol. Liver is a detox organ, and if your body shuttles fructose straight to your liver first, then that implies fructose is a toxic substance that needs to be quarantined and detoxed.

- Fructose is half of table sugar, and table sugar spikes your insulin and blood sugar to high levels.
- Fructose increases uric acid in your blood. Uric acid causes painful diseases like gout.
- Fructose increases your cholesterol levels. Cholesterol clogs your arteries and is damaging to your heart.
- Fructose makes people fat by causing problems with carbohydrate metabolism. When you have problems with carbohydrate metabolism, you can't burn off the carbohydrates you eat.
- Fructose can cause fatty liver because fructose is processed by your liver. If your liver is overloaded, then it turns the fructose into fat. That fat piles up in your liver and causes nonalcoholic fatty liver disease.

Let's take a look at what's really going on with each negative statement about fructose.

Fructose goes straight to your liver:

It is said that the majority of fructose goes to your liver, and that is true[11]. Your liver has the largest ability to use fructose, and that is a good thing, not a bad thing.

Why is it a good thing? Fructose goes straight to your liver because fructose is fuel for your liver, and you want your liver fueled up and happy[12]. Your liver is vital to your health, and if your liver is not healthy, then there is a good chance the rest of your body will not be healthy either[12,13,14]. Your liver is the primary detox center for your body, and it takes in negative substances to get rid of them.

Your liver also stores a significant amount of carbohydrates as a backup source. If you skip a meal, or are asleep and not eating, then your blood sugar will run low[15]. When your blood sugar runs low, your liver comes to the rescue and releases its stored carbohydrates. If you've ever woken up in the middle of the night for no reason, it may be because your liver is low on carbohydrates, and your body is releasing stress hormones like adrenaline and cortisol to increase your blood sugar. Adrenaline is one of the fight or flight hormones, and stress can wake you up and keep you alert. Keeping your liver fueled up can help prevent these midnight stress wakeups[16].

Your brain and body rely on your liver to get extra energy from carbohydrates when you are running low. Your liver is not the only place you can store carbohydrates though, as you can also store carbohydrates in your muscles. However, the carbohydrates in your muscles are not used for keeping your blood sugar regulated, but are mainly used for exercise.

It's the carbohydrates stored in your liver that keep your blood sugar controlled and your stress hormones low. Because of this, giving your liver enough carbohydrates is a sound strategy for maintaining a healthy body. Fructose is a helpful tool for supplying your liver with fuel because fructose is transported directly to your liver first, and gives it the energy it needs to stay strong[11]. A strong liver is a happy liver, and a happy liver helps detox your body and keep your blood sugar regulated.

Fructose spikes your insulin:

Many people casually say that fructose will spike your insulin levels, but the truth is that fructose hardly has any effect on your insulin levels at all. Fructose does not stimulate insulin release; even protein increases insulin more than fructose.

For example, if you take a look at the glycemic index of fructose, it's 19[17]. That's even less than a carrot[18]. Then compare that to the glycemic index of a baked white potato. The potato's number is 111, almost 5 times as high as fructose[18]. The reality is that fructose has virtually no impact on insulin[17].

Fructose spikes your blood sugar:

It is often said that fructose will spike your blood sugar, but that is not true. Studies show that fructose has a minimal effect on blood sugar[19]. In fact, research illustrates that if people with diabetes replace the same quantity of carbohydrates as they are eating now with fructose, that fructose improves their long term blood sugar levels— without affecting their insulin[20]. Eating fructose before a meal can even reduce the increase in blood sugar of that meal[21].

Fructose increases your uric acid:

Yes, fructose does increase uric acid, and that can sound alarming because uric acid can cause gout. However, what you may not know is that uric acid is one of the most powerful antioxidants in our bodies. Uric acid is such a powerful antioxidant that scientists believe it was likely a key part of our evolution in becoming humans[22].

Uric acid increased human's life spans, and decreased our susceptibility to cancer[23]. Uric acid also helps protect against damage to cells when unstable fats are used for energy[23]. In short, uric acid is a powerful protector in our bodies, and if fructose increases uric acid, it could be a positive thing for your lifespan and your resistance to cancer. Of course, too much of anything can cause problems, and if uric acid crystallizes in your body it can cause gout. But you can also get gout if your kidneys don't produce enough uric acid[24]. Again, a balance is needed. Not too little, not too much.

Fructose increases your cholesterol:

Fructose can elevate your cholesterol, and it is important to understand that increased cholesterol, to a point, can be beneficial[25]. Cholesterol promotes health and vitality in reasonable quantities because cholesterol can be an antioxidant in your body[26]. Cholesterol is also the building block to many important steroid hormones[27]. If you want to create healthy hormones, which help build your body, you will need enough cholesterol to do so[27]. Low levels of cholesterol can create problems just like high levels can[25]. Again, as with most things, a balance is needed.

It is reasonably safe to say that cholesterol starts causing problems when it's being created faster than it's being used[28,29]. Many people have high levels because their cholesterol is not being converted to hormones, and therefore cholesterol is "backing up" in their bloodstream[28,29].

It is best to create relatively high levels of cholesterol, and then quickly get rid of that cholesterol by converting it to beneficial hormones. That way, you have an abundant supply of building blocks (cholesterol) and you are actually using those building blocks to create beneficial hormones. If you are making a significant amount of cholesterol, and using that cholesterol, then the levels of cholesterol in your blood can still be within healthy ranges.

How do you make sure you are using your cholesterol to make beneficial hormones, and make sure it's not backing up in your blood? There are many factors involved in the inner workings of cholesterol, but the short answer is you need to make sure you have a healthy metabolism, are eating enough food to support your metabolism, and are keeping your thyroid healthy and getting enough vitamin A. This is because the thyroid hormone, plus vitamin A, plus cholesterol, equals pregnenolone, which is the precursor to beneficial hormones your body needs.

We will explore more about how to get vitamin A and keep your thyroid strong later in this book. But, basically, if your metabolism is burning "hot" and chugging along smoothly, you should have lots of cholesterol available in your bloodstream and be using that cholesterol to create hormones on a consistent basis. If you have extremely high levels of cholesterol, it may be a sign that you are not using the cholesterol available in your bloodstream and it is "backing up."[28,29]

Fructose makes you fat:

Many people will tell you that fructose can make you fat because fructose can damage your metabolism and impair your ability to use carbohydrates for energy. This is not true, and these claims are usually backed up by poorly designed studies. These studies should be largely ignored because of three primary reasons.

Reason 1: Rats do not handle fructose as well as humans.[31]

Reason 2: Researchers often grossly overfeed rats on fructose, with a dose larger than most humans could possibly consume.[30]

Reason 3: Isolated fructose is virtually never found in nature. Fructose is almost always accompanied by glucose, and that is exactly what sugar is, half glucose, half fructose. Studies done with pure fructose are unrealistic and do not apply to real world situations.[31]

Lastly, fructose does not make people fat because the fact is that studies show fructose added to glucose increases total carbohydrate usage as compared to glucose alone[32]. So when you eat glucose and fructose together—like you find in sugar—your ability to use carbohydrates for energy goes up, not down, and that means an increased metabolism.

Fructose causes fatty liver disease:

Some will tell you that because fructose goes straight to your liver, that fructose will turn into fat in your liver. It will cause your liver to accumulate too much fat and that will result in nonalcoholic fatty liver disease.

The fact is that overeating on any food can cause nonalcoholic fatty liver disease, not just fructose[33], but studies show that choline—a B-vitamin found in eggs and liver—can prevent or even reverse a fatty liver[34,35]. Studies have even shown that people who have a genetic variation, and are not able to produce choline, are much more susceptible to getting a fatty liver[36]. Because of this, getting enough choline in your diet is likely more important than avoiding fructose.

It is reasonable to believe that overeating of any kind can result in a fatty liver. But if you have a nutrient rich diet that includes sufficient choline, then you may be protected from fatty liver, regardless of fructose consumption.

Chapter 6

LET'S LOOK AT HONEY

Sugar has gotten a bad reputation in the media. For whatever reason, the facts about sugar have been twisted negatively. However, this seems to only happen when the literal word "sugar" is attached to the information. But what is the closest substance to sugar in nature? Honey.

Honey is basically sugar from bees. Honey is almost identical to white refined sugar, and somehow honey has flown under the radar of the sugar media attacks. Honey has been researched extensively, but it has not attracted the attention of researchers who are motivated to get in the media by attacking sugar. Because honey is almost identical to sugar—but has not received the same media attack—looking at the benefits of honey can also shine some light on the benefits of sugar.

It is important to note that while honey is almost pure glucose and fructose mixed together just like refined table sugar, honey contains some key differences.

What Makes Honey Different?

Honey is the only sweetener that can be stored and used exactly as it is produced in nature. Honey is a complicated biologically created substance with an elaborate chemical composition. Honey is made primarily of glucose and fructose, just like white sugar, but it also contains at least 181 other substances[1,2]. Some of these substances include vitamins, minerals, proteins, complex carbohydrates, free amino acids, enzymes, flavonoids, phenolic acids, antioxidants, volatile compounds, and so on. Some of the more recognizable elements found in honey—however in small amounts—

are salt, calcium, potassium, magnesium, phosphorus, selenium, copper, iron, manganese, chromium, zinc, vitamin C, vitamin K, and vitamins b1, b2, b3, b5, b6, and b9. Of course, the composition of honey is going to change depending on where the hives are located, and what environment the bees interact with.

The highest concentration of substances other than glucose and fructose found in honey are fructooligosaccharides[3]. Fructooligosaccharides compose about 34% of honey and are basically a type of fiber digested by the part of your colon called the cecum. These fructooligosaccharides are known to feed a "friendly" bacteria species called bifidobacteria. When a food feeds friendly bacteria, it is often referred to as a "prebiotic," so because honey can feed good bacteria it can be said that honey is a prebiotic substance.

Fructooligosaccharides are technically a fiber in the "inulin" family. And inulin fiber has been shown to reduce LDL cholesterol in obese patients. It can help increase calcium absorption, as well as possibly magnesium absorption. Studies have also shown that adding six grams of inulin to food can be as filling as 260 extra calories, and help reduce hunger.

Beyond honey having fructooligosaccharides, as mentioned above, honey contains approximately 181 other substances that are yet to be completely understood. And although we don't know everything about the substances in honey, we do know that honey appears to have significant benefits for most people who eat it.

How Does Honey Contain 181 Different Substances?

Those approximately 181 substances are most likely a result of tens of thousands of bees landing on millions of flowers and bringing back little bits of material with them to mix in with the honey. It is that mix of little bits of the environment all condensing into one concentrated source that gives your body exposure to a large part of your environment. With a food that grows in the ground or on a tree, you are getting the environmental factors from that one spot of land. But with honey you are getting little "bites" of millions of bees over a large radius of land[4].

As a result of the local environment essentially being concentrated in a single substance, many people feel that the environmental exposure through honey can help reduce allergies, especially if you eat local honey.

This theory is highly debated, and there is little proof that honey actually helps with allergies, even local honey[5], and although no studies have definitively proved honey helps with allergies, many people do report that it helps them despite the lack of scientific evidence.

While there are many beneficial substances in honey, it is important to note that some of these substances could be contaminants such as pesticides, fuel from cars, farm equipment, or other random small materials that the bees could touch and bring back to the hive[6].

Antioxidant Capacity

Honey contains antioxidants, and it appears that the darker the honey, the more antioxidants it's likely to contain. Researchers have found that humans can be significantly protected from free radical damage by the antioxidants in honey[8]. That means there aren't just antioxidants in honey, but that the antioxidants are biologically available, which is an important distinction.

So now that we understand the key differences between refined white sugar and honey, let's start talking about what good things honey has been shown to do.

Athletic Performance

Athletic performance can be improved with the use of honey and can be a better substitute to options that contain only glucose as their primary ingredient. This has been tested on cyclists who were given a glucose-only gel, and other cyclists who were given honey instead[9]. Both the glucose and honey caused an increase in performance, but the honey produced even better results than glucose. This can be partly due to the fact that honey releases sugar into your blood slower than pure glucose, or even pure sugar. Honey takes longer to digest and has a "slow burn" effect, letting energy "trickle" into your body, which can be beneficial for increasing physical performance, specifically endurance related performance[10].

The slow digesting nature of honey can be attributed to its concentration of fructose combined with complex oligosaccharides carbohydrates, such as maltose, melezitose, palatinose, trehalose, raffinose, isomaltose, maltulose, maltotriose, panose, erlose, turanose, gentiobiose and cellobiose. It is because of this slowly digesting effect that some researchers believe honey can have an anti-diabetic effect[21].

Anemia

Honey has also been found to help with anemia because of its ability to build blood volume and red blood cells[11]. In addition, honey also appears to be able to help with building immunity by increasing production of antibodies[12].

Tooth Decay

Many people claim that sugar can contribute to tooth decay. While this could be true with sugar, it appears that honey can do the exact opposite. Honey with high levels of antibacterial properties can actually reduce the risk of cavities[13]. Plaque and gingivitis can also be reduced by eating honey[14]. Honey can even be less likely to produce cavities than fruit juice[15]. No one knows exactly why honey prevents or produces less tooth and gum decay than other sugar-like substances, but some theories discuss the antibacterial properties as well as the trace amounts of colloidal calcium, fluoride, and phosphorus.

Stomach Issues

Ulcers and other digestive issues can be prevented by the use of honey[16]. Ulcers are often caused by a bacteria called Helicobacter pylori, and honey is able to help prevent that bacteria from growing, or potentially kill it off when it's already become a problem. Due to honey's natural acidity, and small levels of hydrogen peroxide, it has the potential to inhibit some pathogens[17].

Wound healing can also be increased by the use of topical honey, even in wounds that were not healing quickly with other treatments[20]. This is probably due to the antimicrobial properties in honey, as well as creating a sticky barrier that protects against contaminants making contact with the wound.

Eye Health

Eye health can also be improved through the use of topical honey, especially in the treatment of "pink eye" or in the inflammation of the cornea, or the eyelids[18]. Specifically, applying a drop of honey under the lower eyelid can have the most benefit, even if that honey is diluted by a 50% water mixture.

Blood Sugar and Cholesterol Influence

Honey can also help reduce overall blood glucose levels, and cholesterol levels compared to other sweeteners[19]. Therefore, honey as a sweetener choice can be especially beneficial if your goal is to lower and stabilize your blood sugar and cholesterol levels. This lowering of cholesterol is most likely due to honey's ability to increase the active thyroid hormone called T3 because any carbohydrate is actually able to help increase T3 concentrations, especially fructose, which honey contains a great deal of[22,23,24,25]. When T3 increases, it can convert cholesterol into other beneficial substances, such as hormones. When cholesterol is converted for beneficial purposes, it can lower your overall cholesterol number[26,27].

Metabolic Syndrome, Diabetes and Obesity

There are even some researchers that claim—although with unpublished research—that honey cannot induce metabolic syndrome. Metabolic syndrome is also said to be responsible for many chronic health issues, such as obesity, and Diabetes 2. In addition to honey possibly not being able to cause metabolic syndrome, it can also help prevent overeating because honey can potentially help modulate appetite-regulating hormones and make you feel fuller longer[28,29].

With all of these potential benefits of honey, ranging from tasting great, to helping boost athletic performance, reducing cholesterol, and helping to prevent diabetes and obesity, honey is certainly not a bad food choice for most people. In fact, honey seems to be much more beneficial than it is harmful in almost all cases.

And knowing that honey is essentially the same substance as refined sugar, with the exception of the trace minerals, antioxidants, and antimicrobial properties, many of the same benefits can be applied to sugar, especially in the categories of athletic performance, anemia, blood sugar, and cholesterol. But because there are additional benefits to honey, as compared to refined sugar, the additional benefits of honey highlight that unprocessed sugars are likely a better choice for most people.

Chapter 7

WHAT ABOUT DIABETES 2?

It is commonly believed that sugar is largely responsible for Diabetes type 2. The media has certainly blamed Diabetes type 2 on sugar. But is the media right? Is it the sugar? Before we come to any conclusions, let's dig a little deeper. What is Diabetes 2? How do we define it? And how do we know when people have it?

Before we get into the fundamentals of The First Diet, we must understand Diabetes 2. Why must we understand Diabetes 2? Because getting your carbohydrate metabolism running as well as possible is one of the main goals of The First Diet.

Diabetes 2 is the exact opposite of a healthy carbohydrate metabolism and therefore it will show us the reverse of what we want to achieve. Seeing the flipside of a properly functioning carbohydrate metabolism will be helpful in understanding what makes a robust carbohydrate metabolism. In addition, Diabetes 2 is so common in our modern world it is critical to understand how Diabetes 2 happens and what can go wrong, so we can avoid these problems and get things right instead.

Remember, the term "blood sugar" really means blood glucose, and Diabetes 2 is basically, at its core, elevated blood sugar levels[1]. There are a few ways doctors measure to see if you have elevated blood sugar levels, such as doing a fasted blood glucose test, a random blood glucose test, an oral glucose tolerance test, or a measure of your average blood glucose over 23 months with a glycated hemoglobin test.

Doctors are basically looking to see if you have higher than normal blood sugar levels on a consistent basis. If you do, then you likely have an inability to metabolize your blood sugar. That means you have too much blood sugar floating around in your veins all the time, and that's not a good thing. And that "not good thing" is called Diabetes 2.

To understand what may cause elevated blood sugar, let's look at what can cause blood sugar to go up and down. There are countless factors that influence blood sugar levels, but here it is at a basic level.

Your blood sugar goes up when you eat, especially carbohydrates, and it goes up when you release stress hormones for energy (think fear or fasting).

Your blood sugar goes down when you metabolize carbohydrates without replacing them. Or it goes down when you produce insulin to help put that sugar into your cells for use or storage.

If the systems that influence blood sugar moving up and down are not working correctly, then what are some potential causes for that happening? We are going to rely heavily on the knowledge we gained in the earlier chapter on carbohydrate metabolism here.

Cause number 1: Glucose gets into your cells, but then isn't used fully.

In this case, the unused glucose gets turned into lactate, pushed back into your bloodstream and then converted back into glucose again through your liver[2]. That basically means that glucose gets into your cell and gets bumped right back out again. If this happens, it indicates your cells aren't using the carbohydrates you eat—sugar or otherwise—and the excess is backing up into your bloodstream. That causes elevated blood glucose.

If this is the case, then you are producing enough insulin for the glucose to get into your cells, and your cells are accepting the insulin, but something on the inside of your cells is not working. The mitochondria inside your cells may not be using the sugar correctly, and that means your mitochondria are possibly damaged. Mitochondria are needed to fully use glucose, otherwise that glucose turns into lactate. Also, enough oxygen is needed to fully process the glucose. For example, if you're working out hard, you can produce lactic acid because of the shortage of oxygen caused by exercise. When there isn't enough oxygen to use glucose, that glucose gets transformed to lactic acid instead of being used for energy.

Number 2: Glucose never gets into your cells.

In this case, there may not be enough insulin produced to shove the glucose into your cells. If this is true, there is a good chance you have a fatty liver and fatty pancreas[3,4]. Your insulin is produced by your pancreas, and if your pancreas is overburdened with fat, it may not be able to produce enough insulin. Therefore, if you aren't producing adequate amounts of insulin, then you probably won't be getting enough glucose into your cells.

Or maybe the glucose isn't getting into your cells because your cells are insulin resistant. In this scenario you would be producing enough insulin, but your cells would not be using that insulin. If insulin isn't recognized by your cells, then insulin can't bring glucose into your cells to be turned into energy. And if glucose is not able to enter your cells, then it will be backing up in your bloodstream and elevating your blood sugar levels.

So what are some potential solutions for fixing the issues of Diabetes 2? Let's tackle them by the two different scenarios laid out above, one being that glucose gets into your cells but isn't used fully, and two being that glucose never gets into your cells to begin with.

If glucose gets into your cells but isn't used fully, then it is likely that you have damaged mitochondria, or you may be eating too much glucose for your body to use. If your mitochondria are damaged, many people diagnosed with Diabetes 2 take a drug called metformin which is thought to help multiply and possibly repair mitochondria. And it does seem to help some people get Diabetes 2 under control. Exercise can also help create more undamaged mitochondria.

In addition, eating to support your mitochondria would be a good idea, and that basically means eating a balanced diet, trying your best to get all of your vitamins and minerals from real food sources, and also getting balanced amounts of carbohydrates, protein and fat. Shortly we will explore how The First Diet works and can help you construct a diet that can help you do this.

If you are getting glucose into your cells but then not using that glucose inside your cells, and your mitochondria are not damaged, then you may simply be eating too much food. In that case, it is reasonable to assume that someone would be able to self-diagnose in this department, but it's fairly safe to say that if you're already overweight and are still gaining weight, and you have been diagnosed with Diabetes 2, eating too much may be a significant part of the issue. Cutting back on your calories could have a positive effect.

What about if glucose never gets into your cells in the first place?

In this situation you probably are not producing enough insulin to get the glucose into your cells. That may be due to having a fatty pancreas. If you do have a fatty pancreas, which is overburdened and unable to produce enough insulin, then it could be a good idea to eat less and/or exercise more. Basically, if you want to lose fat on your internal organs—like your pancreas and liver—you'll need to go on a fat loss plan. If you are able to lose fat on your body, then at some point you will start to lose fat on your pancreas. That fat loss may help your pancreas start to produce enough insulin again.

Alternatively, if you are producing enough insulin, but you still are unable to get glucose into your cells, then you may be insulin resistant. That means your cells just don't recognize insulin very well any longer. One of the best ways to increase insulin sensitivity is to exercise more, and to eat a balanced diet, like we'll discuss in a later chapter.

Some early symptoms of Diabetes type 2 include: frequent infections that heal slowly, fatigue, hunger, increased thirst, increased urination, blurred vision, erectile dysfunction, pain or numbness in the hands or feet, mood swings, and irritability. Diabetes type 2 can even cause a reduction in brain volume[5]. In fact, Alzheimer's disease is now being thought of by some researchers as a form of Diabetes of the brain[6]. This conclusion is made because Diabetes is defined by the inability to use blood glucose efficiently, and the brains of people with Alzheimer's disease are also unable to use blood glucose efficiently. Eventually, this can lead to brain impairment, shrinkage, and Alzheimer's disease[6].

Ultimately, this all is a complicated way of saying that Diabetes type 2 means your body isn't using glucose well. And if you're not using glucose well, then you probably need to lose some fat, exercise more, and eat a balanced, pro-metabolic diet—like what you'll find in The First Diet.

Essentially, Diabetes type 2 is the result of an unstable metabolic system that is not able to handle glucose properly. In order to prevent this issue, or fix it, we must stabilize our body's metabolism. And on the topic of stability, let's talk about fats.

Chapter 8

THE FAT CHAPTER

There are three primary types of fats that you can eat: saturated fat, monounsaturated fat, and polyunsaturated fat. It is important to note that the fat you eat is almost always stored as fat in your fat cells, or it can be stored inside your muscles[1,2].

When you eat fat, you can be pretty certain it's going to be stored as fat inside your body, at least temporarily. You can store virtually unlimited amounts of fat inside your body. If your fat cells can't hold any more fat, they will often create more fat cells to allow you to store even more fat[3].

Because the fat you eat is transferred from your digestive system to your bloodstream and then stored, it is still the same type of fat that you ate. So if you eat saturated fat, you will store saturated fat; if you eat monounsaturated fat, you will store monounsaturated fat; and if you eat polyunsaturated fat you will store polyunsaturated fat[2,3]. As the saying goes, you are what you eat.

Another way of putting this is: If you eat mostly polyunsaturated fat, eventually, most of the fat on your body will be polyunsaturated. If you eat mostly monounsaturated fat, eventually, most of the fat on your body will be monounsaturated. And if you eat mostly saturated fat, eventually, most of the fat on your body will be saturated.

This is true for almost all animals that have one stomach. But "ruminant" animals like cows and sheep have four compartment stomachs. What is unique about four compartment stomachs is that they convert over 90% of the unsaturated fats they eat into saturated fats[4]. That makes the fat in beef and lamb mostly saturated, and monounsaturated. This is important, and we will get to why in a minute. But first we need to know the differences in the types of fat you can eat and why it matters.

Saturated Fat:

You'll generally know a fat is saturated when it's solid at room temperature and gets hard in the refrigerator. Good sources of saturated fat are coconut oil, butter and fat from animals like beef and lamb.

Saturated fat is extremely stable compared to other fats, and will stay fresh much longer than other fats without going "rancid." This is mainly due to its chemical structure being more secure, which is reflected physically by its "hardness." You'll also notice that if you touch foods with high saturated fat contents, like butter or coconut oil, they will instantly melt on your finger. So, when they become the temperature of your body, they will not harden up, and therefore will not harden up in your body, or your arteries as long as you are alive.

Because of saturated fat's stable nature, it is less prone to being damaged by free radicals, and because of that, it could be considered a natural antioxidant because it does not oxidize as easily as the other types of fats.

Common sources of saturated fat are butter, coconut oil, cheese, milk, and cream. Beef and lamb fat are also about half saturated.

Monounsaturated Fat:

Monounsaturated fat is liquid at room temperature, but will also harden in the refrigerator. The highest concentration of monounsaturated fat you will likely encounter is olive oil, and avocados have a fairly concentrated quantity as well. Monounsaturated fat is found in most animal and plant fats. You'll see significant amounts of these fats in beef, pork, lamb, chicken, etc.

Monounsaturated fat is not quite as stable as saturated fat, and that's physically reflected by its liquid and "pourable" nature. It is still stable, but will oxidize and "go rancid" faster than saturated fat. However, monounsaturated fat is still significantly resistant to free radicals in your body, and it's also another good "antioxidant" in the sense that it is resistant to oxidative damage.

Common sources of monounsaturated fats are olive oil and avocados. Beef and lamb fat is also about half monounsaturated fat.

Polyunsaturated Fat: (Also known as omega-6 and omega-3 fatty acids.)

Polyunsaturated fat is liquid at room temperature and liquid in the refrigerator. The highest concentration of polyunsaturated fat you will likely encounter is in vegetable and seed oils like corn oil, soy oil, canola oil, peanut oil, flax seed oil, and sunflower seed oil. Omega-3, like in fish oil, is also a polyunsaturated fat.

Polyunsaturated fat is additionally found in animals that are fed these types of fats. For example, many animals are fed soy and flax. As we discussed earlier, for many animals, including humans (with the exception of animals with four stomachs that are meant to eat grass, like cows and sheep), the fat they eat is the fat they store. For animals like chickens and pigs, if they eat a significant quantity of soy, then the polyunsaturated fat from the soy will be reflected in the structure of the animal's tissues. This works the same way as when farmers make "omega-3 rich eggs" by feeding their chickens flax seed because the omega-3 from the flax seed makes it into the chicken's bodies, and then into the eggs. Animals like chickens and pigs that have been fed mostly polyunsaturated fat will have significant amounts of polyunsaturated fat when you put them on your dinner plate. And then when you eat that meat, you will have more polyunsaturated fat stored on your body.

Polyunsaturated fats are the least stable of the fats you will eat, and are likely to be oxidized and "go rancid" even before you eat them. Polyunsaturated fats are also prone to be damaged by free radicals in your body. This susceptibility to being damaged by free radicals and oxidized in your body is because of their chemical structure.

The "poly" in the name polyunsaturated is there because "poly" means "many," and polyunsaturated fats have many "weak spots" in their chemical structure called "methylene groups." These polyunsaturated fats are also much more likely to have something called "lipid peroxidation" happen to them inside your body, which can result in cellular damage.

Because of polyunsaturated fat's ability to oxidize much easier than the other two types of fats discussed, they could be classified as a "pro-oxidant" instead of an "antioxidant." Some of these fats are necessary for overall health, but relying on them heavily for a calorie source could be problematic in the long term.

You will find saturated and monounsaturated fats naturally occurring closer to tropical environments, and polyunsaturated fats naturally occurring further away from tropical environments. For example, coconuts are mostly made of saturated fats and coconuts naturally grow smack dab in the middle of the tropics. Avocados are mostly monounsaturated fats, and they also naturally grow in the tropics, but further away from the equator than coconuts. Omega-3 polyunsaturated rich fish, like salmon, naturally swim around in the freezing cold water of Alaska—almost as far away from the tropics and equator as possible.

This makes biological sense, as the further away from the tropics the more polyunsaturated fats show up in nature, and the closer to the tropics the more saturated fats show up. What happens to saturated fats when you put them in the refrigerator? They harden up. Butter is soft outside the refrigerator, and when you put it inside the refrigerator it firms up into a solid brick. If a salmon was made of saturated fat, as soon as it hit the freezing waters of Alaska, it would stiffen up and be unable to swim. But these fish are made up of a significant amount of polyunsaturated fats, which don't solidify in cold temperatures. If you put fish oil in the refrigerator, it will stay liquid, and that's exactly what a salmon requires. The salmon needs to stay liquid at significantly cold temperatures in order to be able to move around.

But you are not a salmon, and you do not swim around in freezing cold water all day. In fact, your body is designed to maintain a tropical-like environment inside of you 24 hours a day, 7 days a week. Your body should be 98.6 degrees no matter what the temperature is outside. And if your internal body temperature goes too far outside of that 98.6 degree range, you could die. Your body does not like to get much colder or hotter than 98.6 degrees. So what happens if you eat a lot of cold water salmon?

Firstly, if you eat a lot of salmon, your body will begin to be made up of the same fat that the salmon is made of—just like we talked about earlier. The fat you eat is the fat you store. And what happens when fish oil is left out at 98.6 degrees? That's right, it begins to oxidize and spoil.

Of course, your body has many different processes that help keep your body from oxidizing—you may know of some of these as "antioxidants," but your body can only keep up with so much oxidation[5]. Polyunsaturated fats, like those found in vegetable oil and salmon, oxidize very easily as compared to monounsaturated and saturated fats[6]. So the more polyunsaturated fats you are made of, the more oxidation you are prone to having inside of your body, and the harder your body has to fight to keep from "going rancid."

And yes, your body can put up a good fight, but you don't want your body to fight consistently harder than it has to. Your body has enough to do with just keeping you alive, regulating your blood sugar, maintaining your brain function, fending off pathogens, and incomprehensibly more. Adding increased oxidation to the equation only makes things more difficult and stressful.

Like we discussed earlier, polyunsaturated fats are prone to lipid peroxidation[7]. Lipid peroxidation is basically when a polyunsaturated fat gets hit by a free radical and then causes a chain reaction. Because "poly" means "many," polyunsaturated fats have "many" spots where a free radical can hit, and then break a weak spot. When a free radical breaks a weak spot, the break can create another free radical, which hits another weak spot, and the chain reaction can continue. The more polyunsaturated fats you are made of, the more chance the chain reaction can keep going for longer and longer.

You can think of polyunsaturated fats as a loaded mouse trap, and a free radical as a ping pong ball. When you drop the ping pong ball on the ground, the more mouse traps you have loaded on the floor, the more chance many mouse traps will go off from just one ball dropping.

Once dropped, the ball will bounce and hit one mouse trap, then the trap will snap, and throw the ping pong ball into the air, fall, and land on another loaded mouse trap. That trap will snap and throw the ball into the air. The "bounce snap" cycle will repeat until the ball misses a trap, or until there are no more traps to snap. The longer the chain reaction goes on for, the more cell damage can occur. This damage can happen to your cell membranes and your mitochondria, which then can impair your ability to use glucose, like we talked about earlier with Diabetes 2[8].

Common sources of polyunsaturated fats are vegetable oils like soy oil, corn oil, canola oil, sunflower oil and fish oil. Animal sources include cold water fish like salmon, and pigs and chickens that are given polyunsaturated fats as feed on their farms. Soybean feed is common and contributes to the polyunsaturated content of these animals.

If we want maximum health, energy, and longevity, we should do our best to avoid excessive oxidation and free radical damage. One step in that direction is to minimize polyunsaturated fats, and replace them with monounsaturated and saturated fats, the same good fats that naturally grow in tropical environments and stay stable at 98.6 degrees.

Completely removing polyunsaturated fats is not realistic, and not advisable. Almost every fat source contains at least a small amount of omega-6 or omega-3 fats. But the "essential" nature of polyunsaturated fats is largely a scientific debate, and becoming truly deficient in polyunsaturated fats is likely impossible to do. Because polyunsaturated fats are virtually everywhere in our modern society, there is no need to actively seek out polyunsaturated sources. Instead, it can be a better idea to minimize their consumption. Relying on monounsaturated and saturated fats will still give most people enough polyunsaturated fats, because virtually no food is devoid of omega-6 or omega-3.

To recap so far, we know that humans evolved in the tropical environment of Africa where saturated fat and sugar were commonplace. We know that inside our bodies we are bathing in a tropical environment, and any food we eat, we are exposing to that environment. Because of this, we want to give our bodies the foods that helped us become human and the foods that help stabilize our bodies. Two of those foods are sugar and saturated fat. Sugar gives our brains and bodies energy. We discussed the benefits of fructose in sugar, and we now know the advantages of the chemical stability of saturated fats. Next we will discuss how protein fits into this picture.

Chapter 9

PROTEIN

You can store the fat you eat in your fat cells, and you can store the carbohydrates you eat in your muscles and liver. But, unlike fat and carbohydrates, there is no official storage cell for protein; however, protein makes up the majority of the structure of your body. Protein is used either to repair or maintain your body's functions, and protein is also used to build new structures in your body, like more muscle. In addition, protein can be turned into carbohydrates if your body does not have enough carbohydrates to use when it needs more blood sugar. The process of converting protein into carbohydrates is called gluconeogenesis. Using gluconeogenesis on a consistent basis to create carbohydrates can be stressful to your body over time[1].

Protein can come from plants or animals. People argue that some proteins are "incomplete," and while that is true, it does seem that it's possible to build muscle and other tissue with both plant and animal proteins. However, diversifying your protein intake can be a good strategy.

Why could it be smart to diversify your protein consumption? Some amino acids are found in certain types of proteins, while others are left out. And not all amino acids are necessarily beneficial in large amounts.

One amino acid that is mostly found in animal connective tissues, like skin, and tendons, is glycine. Glycine is not present in significant quantities in muscle meat, like steaks and chicken breasts. Plant proteins also are lacking in glycine, so if you want to include glycine in your diet, you will have to eat animals "nose to tail," and that means being more like our tropical ancestors, and not just selecting the steak from a cow, and the chicken breast from the chicken.

Glycine is an important amino acid that is often neglected due to the fact that connective tissues are not a common part of modern diets any longer. The amino acid glycine can help with your liver health, and your liver's ability to detox[2]. Without glycine, you are probably not giving your liver everything it needs to be most efficient, and we already know that a healthy liver is a key element to a healthy body.

In order to get glycine from these animals, our tropical ancestors likely ate the feet, skin, and other not-so-appetizing bits of the animals they hunted. Don't worry, though: There are many ways to get glycine in your diet without having to resort to horrendous sounding meals. Bone broths or gelatin powder are two easy and modern options. We will get into more detail about this in later chapters.

In our modern diets, two common amino acids are tryptophan and cysteine. These are found in muscle meat, like steaks and chicken breast. Both of these amino acids are essential to your body, but too much of anything can become harmful. If you are relying on muscle meat as your primary protein source, then you may be getting more of these amino acids than you need.

Tryptophan is the only known carcinogenic amino acid[3]. And cysteine can temporarily inhibit your thyroid[4]. Neither of these amino acids are bad in-and-of-themselves, but it's about balance. This is part of why not relying on one protein source alone, and making sure to diversify, is most likely a beneficial approach.

Protein is essential to your health, and your body's ability to repair damage, heal wounds, build muscle, and protein is very helpful to your liver as well[5]. Getting enough protein is essential, but also diversifying your protein sources, such as eating connective tissues as well as muscle meat, can be a smart strategy.

Up to this point in the book we have covered why protein, saturated fats, and sugar can be beneficial substances. But that's not the whole picture because you can't live on protein, sugar and saturated fat alone. There are many more aspects to nutrition and a great number of those aspects are in the vitamins and minerals of our foods. We will discuss vitamins and minerals right after we talk about a toxic human condition that plagues us all—stress.

Chapter 10

STRESS

Now that we have a better understanding of the primary food classifications, protein, carbohydrates, fat, and their major sub-classifications, let's move on to another important topic: stress. Some stress you can feel in your body, and some stress just runs in the background unnoticed. Chronically stressed people are less healthy, age faster, and have a lower quality of life[1,2,3,4]. Reducing stress is one of the most important things you can do for your health.

Why is stress important for nutrition? There are many reasons why, but there are two primary forms of stress that we'll talk about in this book. Number one is physical stress due to nutritional deficiencies. Number two is psychological stress that originates from your mind.

There are entire industries built around alleviating mental stress, and The First Diet will not be able to cover how to deal with these cognitive stressors in detail. If you are interested in quickly knocking down this type of stress, the best book on the topic I have found is called *The Myth of Stress* by Andrew Bernstein.

In the book, Andrew explores the idea that stress is not caused by our circumstances— stress is caused by our thoughts about our circumstances. For example, a hungry tiger could be right behind you, right now, but if you didn't know about the tiger, you couldn't be stressed about it. However, if you turned around and suddenly saw that tiger right next to you— you would be instantly stressed.

The tiger was behind you the entire time, but you were not stressed until your brain registered the thought. But let's say the tiger is your pet, and you know it's a friendly animal, but you still don't know it's behind you. In this case, you turn around, and may be surprised to see your pet tiger, but you are not nearly as stressed. Andrew argues that most psychological stress is caused by how you think about your circumstances, rather than your absolute circumstances. In both our examples the absolute situation is that a tiger is behind you, but you react differently based on your thoughts.

I highly recommend reading the book. It's repetitive in nature, but that repetitiveness is helpful in understanding the topic. Andrew also has some simple ways of knocking down highly stressful thoughts in just minutes. It's not a relaxation technique or anything spiritual or esoteric; Andrew's method forces you to have an "ah ha" moment about your stressful thoughts, and then you can't see those stressful thoughts in the same way again.

Andrew says that mental stress is usually a contraction of thought, just like a contraction of muscle. So if you have an involuntary contracting muscle, you're usually "tight" and you need to stretch it, like in yoga, or get a massage to relax it. Most people hold contracting thoughts, and they could benefit by stretching the opposite way of thinking. Even if you don't believe the opposite thought, just exploring it is like stretching in the other direction.

An example of a contracting or "tight thought" is anything that feels stressful and begins with "I shouldn't" or "I should." If you feel stress related to that thought, then stretching it out could be beneficial. If you don't feel stress about a "should or shouldn't" thought, then it's probably not a big deal, like, "I shouldn't walk out into traffic." You probably would agree with that, and not stress about it.

However, if you think, "I shouldn't have to do all this work." Or, "There shouldn't be this much traffic." Or, "I should have more money." And if you have stress around those thoughts, then they're "contracted" and "tight," so stretching them in the other way could help.

So, how do you stretch the idea? You simply state the opposite thought, and list supporting truths to add weight to the stretch. It can be frustrating to think the opposite of what you are currently thinking, because you'll often disagree with the opposite statement, but that's just the stretching in action.

For example, if you think, "There shouldn't be this much traffic," you state—or preferably write down—the opposite, which would be, "In reality, there should be this much traffic right now."

Then you start listing why there should be this much traffic right now.

Like:

- This is a growing city that doesn't have enough lanes of traffic to support rush hour.
- People really enjoy driving their cars as compared to public transport in my city.
- It's currently rush hour, and this bad traffic happens every day at this time.

Just keep going as long as you reasonably can. Preferably, you also add something that you are personally, and currently, doing to contribute to the problem.

Like:

- And I'm driving in the traffic, in my car, alone, not carpooling, and adding to the issue, too.

Then you go back to the top and see how the original statement feels now.

There's a few more steps, involving exploring feelings around the contracted statement and the opposite statement. But if you're interested, you should read the book.

The second primary way your body can be stressed is physical stress induced by diet. When you are physically stressed, that generally means your body is working hard to keep your system in balance.

Usually this type of stress is reflected in blood sugar control. For example, the fight or flight response increases blood sugar in order to help you run away, or fight if you need to. Or if you are not eating enough, your body will release stress hormones to help keep your blood sugar up, and to keep you alive. So in order to understand physical stress, we need to understand how your body controls your blood sugar. (Are you sensing a theme with how sugar is very important to your health?)

There are many hormones and other substances that influence blood sugar control, and no one understands them all. There are also likely many more elements that we have yet to discover that play a part in blood sugar regulation. That being said, in the interest of practical application, and understanding the big picture of what we know today, let's talk about the primary hormones you can potentially influence through diet, and what they can do to your blood sugar levels.

Here are the major hormones that influence blood sugar that you should probably care most about. All of these are important to health, and none of them are bad in isolation.

1) Insulin

Insulin can have many positive effects in your body. But right now, we're going to focus on the effect insulin plays on your blood sugar.

Insulin lowers blood sugar. Why does insulin lower blood sugar? Because insulin helps take the sugar in your bloodstream (glucose) and put it into your cells. Once it's in your cells, it's not in your blood any longer, therefore lowering your blood sugar.

What are some foods that increase your insulin levels?

Both carbohydrates and protein will raise insulin levels. Protein can also cause a rise in insulin just as much or more than carbohydrates. It appears that insulin is not only helpful in getting glucose into your cell, but it also helps in protein synthesis, and building muscle.

So it stands to reason that if you eat carbohydrates, then your blood sugar can go up, and then the insulin can take it back down again. If you eat protein alone, then your insulin levels will go up, and your blood sugar will go down. If that decrease is too much, then your body will need to rely on other hormones to bring up your blood sugar again. Those hormones are often glucagon, cortisol, and adrenaline. If you do not want to risk releasing more cortisol or adrenaline than necessary, it could be a good idea to eat protein with carbohydrates together. Carbohydrates eaten with protein can help regulate your blood sugar more smoothly and help keep blood sugar from going too low.

Generally, a 1:1 or 1:2 ratio of protein to carbohydrates is a good idea. For example, if you are eating 20 grams of protein, then eating 20-40 grams of carbohydrates with that protein could help keep your blood sugar stable—without relying excessively on stress hormones.

2) Glucagon

Like any other hormone, glucagon does many things in your body, but for the purpose of understanding blood sugar regulation, we can simply say that glucagon helps increase blood sugar. Glucagon is almost the "opposite" of insulin, and insulin and glucagon are often said to "oppose" each other.

It seems that whenever your blood sugar dips down to a certain threshold, glucagon will swoop in to help raise blood sugar back up again. Glucagon helps increase blood sugar by releasing stored glycogen, and glucagon can also help convert protein into carbohydrates.

In addition, it also appears that when glucagon increases in your body, cortisol, adrenaline, and other stress hormones are not far behind. Glucagon does not work alone in most cases.

3) Cortisol

Cortisol also performs many functions in your body. As with most things, too little is bad, and so is too much.

Cortisol's effect on blood sugar is to raise it. Cortisol often increases blood sugar by converting protein into glucose in your body. Cortisol can do this through the protein you eat, or it can grab protein from your own muscles and use that for raising blood sugar as well.

If your blood sugar is low, glucagon and cortisol will often be released find protein to turn into sugar. If you decide to stop eating carbohydrates, or if you're not eating enough calories, then your blood sugar will most likely dip down to a point where your body needs more.

When your blood sugar hits this low point (you often won't feel this happen[5]), cortisol will jump in and take the protein you are eating and turn that back into carbohydrates, a process called gluconeogenesis. However, if you have lots of stored carbohydrates in your liver and muscles, then your reliance on cortisol should go down.

If you want to avoid cortisol "eating your protein" and turning it back into carbohydrates, it is advisable to eat carbohydrates with protein in the 1:1 or 1:2 ratio talked about previously.

4) Adrenaline

Adrenaline is often referred to as the "fight or flight" hormone, and as with the rest of your hormones, it performs many functions.

Adrenaline raises your blood sugar, and primarily does this by releasing stored carbohydrates (glycogen) in your muscles and liver. Adrenaline can be good when you need it in emergency situations, but it is generally recognized that "running on adrenaline" most of the day can be unhealthy long-term.

When blood sugar gets low enough, just like cortisol, adrenaline will most likely be released to free up stored muscle and liver glycogen in order to raise blood sugar. If you want to avoid excessive adrenaline release, eating adequate carbohydrates is one way to possibly reduce the release of adrenaline.

Unlike insulin and cortisol, people often physically experience the effects of adrenaline. Adrenaline can feel good to many people; it may give them a surge of energy and a sensation of focus. Some people, however, feel bad with adrenaline. Those people will often experience anxiety, heart palpitations, clammy hands, and other adverse reactions. If a low-carb or low-calorie diet gives you energy, it is likely due to an adrenaline surge that's trying to keep you alive.

A synthetic version of adrenaline, called ephedrine, has been sold as a weight loss and energy supplement. It is now illegal to sell as a weight loss supplement, due to its potentially harmful side effects.

Many people have said that if you want six-pack abs, those abs are not made in the gym, they're made in the kitchen. Basically, they're saying you can't out-exercise a bad diet. While that's probably true, there may be another side to that story. You may not be able to out-eat a stressful life. It appears that no matter what you eat, you cannot completely control the release of these types of "stress hormones" like cortisol and adrenaline through diet.

If you are stressed-out, you're probably releasing a combination of stress hormones that no food can completely control. At the same time, there is probably some truth to "stress eating" and "comfort foods," as foods high in sugar can potentially help inhibit these hormones.

The best way to control these hormones is probably through a combination of a proper diet with enough carbohydrates, relaxation, and practices like what are found in the book *The Myth of Stress*.

But getting enough sugar, carbohydrates, diversifying your protein, making sure your fats are saturated or monounsaturated and avoiding stress is not enough. Next we need to talk about vitamins and minerals.

Chapter 11

VITAMINS AND MINERALS

Vitamins and minerals are essential to life, and getting enough of them is one of the keys to not only surviving but thriving. There are more forms of vitamins and minerals than we can ever hope to go into here, and more forms are being discovered on a consistent basis. The good thing is that most of the essential vitamins and minerals appear to be identified, and well-understood.

It is understandable if you want to skip this chapter, as this chapter will not tell you exactly how to use The First Diet for yourself. However, I highly recommend you read through this chapter if you want to understand why The First Diet works so uniquely. This chapter will open your eyes to the complexity of vitamins and minerals, and The First Diet's ability to easily include them all is one of The First Diet's significant advantages.

It is important to get sufficient quantities of vitamins and minerals in your diet, and realizing why you need each can help you assemble the big picture. In addition, reading this chapter will help you discover which foods help maximize your vitamin and mineral intake. In the next chapter we will start to put The First Diet together and show you how certain foods can connect like puzzle pieces and give you the carbs, protein, fat, vitamins and minerals you need. This is important because some diets neglect large chunks of important vitamins and minerals, carbohydrates, fats, or proteins. The First Diet is rounded out, and packs in as much nutrition as realistically possible—simply and elegantly.

The RDA (Recommended Dietary Allowance) or RDI (Recommended Daily Intake) for each vitamin and mineral has been established, and they will be listed in the RDA reference at the end of this book.

The First Diet is not designed to give you exact daily requirements for each vitamin or mineral beyond these recommendations, and there is no realistic way to be perfect on the amounts you get each day. But the RDA is a great place to establish a starting point.

The RDA recommendations appear to be based on good science, and they are likely valid guidelines for most people, whether or not you're on The First Diet. That being said, speaking on a practical level, it can be difficult to get 100% of each recommendation every day by just eating food, and it is debatable if you even need 100% of each vitamin or mineral every single day. Sometimes you might feel better with less, and sometimes you may feel better with more. A great way to see how much of each vitamin and mineral you are getting is to log your daily food intake in a nutritional calculator online. There are many great ones for free.

If you feel like you need more of a specific vitamin for whatever reason, and you need that vitamin "boost" to help solve a health issue or resolve symptoms of a deficiency, then you are almost treating a vitamin as a drug, or a "treatment". In that case, it would be advisable to consult with a medical professional to see what your best options are.

If you feel like you are not getting 100% of the recommended intake of any specific vitamin through your food, and you want to get more of any specific vitamin, supplementation may be a good option.

Even though it may seem like there are too many to process, there are only 6 major classifications of vitamins. There is little point in going into every aspect of each of the vitamins and what exactly they do. Because, knowing everything about each vitamin is almost impossible, as you could probably spend your entire life going down the rabbit hole of each of them. Having said that, there are important things to know about vitamins, and we'll go over the high level significant factors.

Vitamins

1) Vitamin A

Vitamin A is often misunderstood. Many people think they can get it from vegetables like carrots, which contain beta-carotene. Beta-carotene can convert into vitamin A in your body, but many people don't convert beta-carotene into vitamin A efficiently. You need a lot of beta-carotene to make any real amount of vitamin A. Basically, you're probably not going to get a great deal of active vitamin A from plants.

Vitamin A is "fat soluble." That means it can accumulate in your body over time. Because vitamin A can store in your fat, you can get too much vitamin A, and it can be toxic to your body. The likelihood of that happening from actual food, instead of a supplement, is low however—and vitamin A toxicity is not a concern for most people.

Vitamin A's significant high level functions are connected to vision, the immune system, and reproduction. Vitamin A also helps the heart, lungs, kidneys, and skin. Great sources of vitamin A are eggs and liver.

Vitamin A can also help some people reduce the symptoms of acne, and some popular prescription acne medications are made from unnaturally high doses of modified vitamin A. High doses of vitamin A should be monitored by a health professional, as extreme doses can be potentially toxic, as with most substances taken in large doses. Remember, when "mega dosing" with any vitamin or mineral, you are essentially crossing the line from treating them as "foods" and going more into the "using a vitamin or mineral as a drug" category.

Some people believe that liver is a "filter organ" and therefore contains toxins. In truth, the liver is not a filter organ, as it actually removes toxins, and is more like a processing plant than a filter. If you can stomach the taste of liver, and if you get liver from a reputable source you trust, it probably will help your health more than hurt it. Liver is the best source of vitamin A anywhere in nature. Eggs also contain significant quantities of vitamin A.

2) Vitamin B

There are many forms of each type of vitamin, and vitamin B is known for having the most. There are vitamins B1, B2, B3, B5, B6, B7, B9, and B12.

The B vitamins are technically water soluble and shouldn't be able to build up in your body. Technically, you should be able to eat or supplement great quantities of the B vitamins and you'll just urinate them out. That's partly why many vitamin pills cause your urine to be bright yellow.

There is still a bit of debate running that says some B vitamins can build up in your body over time if you consume too much. Some vitamin manufacturers have literally thousands of times the RDA recommended value for B vitamins in their formulas. As with anything, it is a good idea to exercise balance and moderation, and make sure you aren't getting too little or too much of any vitamin.

Liver and eggs are probably your best source of B vitamins. Liver has all of the B vitamins except vitamin B7 (biotin), and eggs do have B7. So together they pretty much cover all your vitamin B bases.

3) Vitamin C

Vitamin C is another water soluble vitamin, so you shouldn't need to worry about "overdosing" on it, within reason. There are not many forms of vitamin C that people generally talk about, with the exception of "ascorbic acid," which is lab-created vitamin C that is often added to foods.

Vitamin C does many things, but its "primary" functions are as an antioxidant; it also helps make collagen, and assists the immune system in working properly. You can usually find vitamin C in citrus fruits like oranges, and other melons and berries like cantaloupe and strawberries. It's basically found in most fruits and vegetables, and is hard to avoid if you are eating a diet with fruits and vegetables, or drinking fruit juice.

4) Vitamin D

Vitamin D is a fat soluble vitamin that interacts with vitamin A, and many experts have recommended a ratio of vitamin A to D of about 5-10:1, meaning that for every IU (International Unit) of vitamin D, you should get 5 or 10 times that much vitamin A. So if you get 3,000 IUs of vitamin A, you would need approximately 300-600 IUs of vitamin D.

This ratio is in line with the RDA guidelines and is most likely recommended because vitamin A and vitamin D seem to "compete" with each other. Too much of one can lead to a lack of the other, so if you're supplementing with vitamin D, you probably want to make sure you are also getting enough vitamin A, and vice versa.

Vitamin D is under a bit of controversy as to whether it should be technically called a vitamin or a hormone. This controversy is partly fueled by the fact that your body can actually make its own vitamin D from the reaction of sunlight on your skin. Regardless of what vitamin D should be classified as, vitamin D is responsible for many things in your body, including helping your body absorb calcium, moving muscles, and carrying messages between your brain and body parts. Your immune system also relies on vitamin D to function at its peak.

How much vitamin D your body will produce varies widely from person to person, depending on multiple factors. Some of these factors include how much time you are out in the sun, how intense the sun's rays are, your own genetic capability to make vitamin D from sunlight, how much skin you are exposing to sunlight, and other influencers. Because of these factors it is challenging to determine how much vitamin D you are making each day.

It is difficult to get enough vitamin D through food alone, so either supplementing with vitamin D3 (which is the most absorbable form) or getting enough sunlight exposure may be important factors when attempting to achieve your vitamin D requirements.

5) Vitamin E

Vitamin E is another fat soluble vitamin, so it can build up in your tissues. However, there seems to be little concern for getting toxic levels in your diet, as it is difficult to get a toxic amount of vitamin E through food.

Vitamin E does many things in your body, but its primary function is to be an antioxidant, which helps protect cells from damage caused by free radicals. It also assists with your immune system, and can help widen blood vessels and prevent blood from clotting. Vitamin E can also assist when cells interact with each other.

Specifically, vitamin E is particularly helpful in preventing something called "lipid peroxidation," which we have previously discussed in the section above about polyunsaturated fats. As a quick summary, "lipid peroxidation" happens when a free radical hits a fat inside your cell membrane, resulting in damage to the cell. Polyunsaturated fats are the most susceptible to this damage due to their chemical composition.

Because vitamin E is important in preventing lipid peroxidation, you will often see greater concentrations of vitamin E with foods that are higher in polyunsaturated fat. This is nature's way of helping keep this polyunsaturated fat from oxidizing too quickly. Some of these foods include sunflower seeds, almonds, and peanuts. Vitamin E can help prevent polyunsaturated fat from oxidizing in your body as well.

Because vitamin E can help prevent lipid peroxidation, it appears that the more polyunsaturated fat you eat in your diet, the more important vitamin E is to your health. The less polyunsaturated fat you eat, the less vitamin E you may need as well. This may be part of why some people believe vitamin E can be good for skin health. Because sunlight can induce free radical damage, and the more polyunsaturated fat you have in your tissues, the more susceptible you can be to having lipid peroxidation happen in your skin. Vitamin E may help prevent some of this sunlight-induced lipid peroxidation damage in your skin cells.

6) Vitamin K

Vitamin K is a unique vitamin, and it's a bit strange because it seems to skip a few letters in the "vitamin alphabet." We have vitamin A, B, C, D, E... and then K. The story behind why vitamin K skips ahead in the "vitamin alphabet" has to do with its discovery in Germany. German scientists found that vitamin K was helpful in coagulation of your blood, and therefore named it vitamin K, after "Koagulation," the German spelling of the word.

Vitamin K is known as the "clotting vitamin," and without it, blood would not clot. Vitamin K also appears to be important in deciding where calcium is transported in your body, and without vitamin K, calcium can be "accidentally" placed in your arteries, and other tissues leading to unwanted calcification and "hardening." If you have enough vitamin K, it appears that calcium is more likely to go to more beneficial locations, such as your bones, instead of possibly contributing to the "hardening of your arteries."

There is no known toxicity issue with vitamin K, especially if you are getting your vitamin K from food sources. However, it is still smart to exercise caution, as vitamin K is a fat soluble vitamin and can build up in your system.

Although there are many forms of every vitamin, there are two major classifications of vitamin K: Vitamin K1 and vitamin K2. Vitamin K1 is mostly found in plants, such as kale. Vitamin K2 is found more in grass-fed animals, and products such as cheese and butter. Grain-fed animals seem to have much less vitamin K in them as compared to grass-fed. Vitamin K2 may be one of the significant benefits of grass-fed animals.

Vitamin K1 is better at blood clotting, and vitamin K2's strength is calcium transport. Vitamin K1 can be converted into K2 inside your body, and K1 can be converted to K2 by bacteria as well, so some fermented foods have a higher concentration of K2 because bacteria is involved in fermentation.

Minerals

Just like vitamins, minerals play a significant role in keeping your body healthy and happy, and certain minerals are required for survival and optimal health.

Calcium

Calcium is the most plentiful mineral found in your body, and that's mostly due to the fact that your bones and teeth contain a great deal of calcium. Calcium is also found in soft tissue, and can be seen in your nerve cells and blood. Calcium can help you build bones and teeth, assists with clotting blood, and sending and receiving nerve signals. It also aids in contracting and relaxing muscles, including your heart. Additionally, calcium can help release hormones and other chemicals. In short, calcium is one of the most important minerals for your body to function correctly, and dietary requirements are significantly high for calcium compared to many other minerals.

If your body needs calcium, and you are not getting enough through diet—because calcium is so important to regulating your day-to-day bodily activities—your body will actually grab calcium from your own bones and put it into your bloodstream for usage.

If your cells do not get enough calcium, they may become "sensitive" to calcium and actually take in more than they need, leading to calcification of certain body tissues, which can be a negative thing for soft tissue. It's almost the exact opposite of what you may think, but the less calcium you eat (within reason) the more your soft tissue seems to calcify. Therefore, the more calcium you eat (within reason) the more calcium should go to the places with the most benefit, like your bones.

As we discussed earlier, how your body uses calcium is highly dependent on how much you eat through diet, as well as the vitamins K, E, D, and A. There is also a balance that goes on with calcium and another mineral called phosphorus. The more phosphorus you eat, the more calcium you may need to help keep your calcium-to-phosphorus balance harmonious. The debate over what ratio is best is still going on, but a good guideline seems to be about 1:1, meaning you should get the same amount of calcium as you do phosphorus. Many people will find that they are getting somewhere around 8 times the amount of phosphorus as calcium in their diet, which may not be optimal.

Why does this ratio matter? This ratio is important because too much phosphorus and too little calcium can increase your parathyroid hormone (PTH.) PTH is responsible for taking calcium out of your bones and putting it into your blood. Too much PTH can weaken your bones over time because it's taking calcium from your bones, and too much PTH can also interfere with your metabolism and lead to an increase in stress hormones as well. It's probably a good idea to get your calcium to phosphorus ratio balanced, at least approximately.

Common foods that are good sources of calcium include dairy, such as, milk, cheese, and yogurt. You can also get calcium from vegetables like spinach or broccoli, but they are not nearly as concentrated as dairy. For example, one cup of milk has about 300 milligrams of calcium, whereas cooked spinach (one of the most concentrated vegetable sources of calcium) only has 240 milligrams of calcium, but spinach's calcium is not well absorbed by your body due to its oxalic acid content[1]. Also, for most people, it is much more difficult to eat a cup of cooked spinach versus drinking a cup of milk.

However, if you are lactose intolerant, you may need to make dietary adjustments, such as eating more calcium-rich vegetables like broccoli or spinach to support your calcium needs. Keep in mind that not all vegetable sources of calcium will be absorbed as well as dairy sources due to oxalic acid (spinach and rhubarb being high sources of oxalic acid) binding to the calcium and inhibiting it from being used by your body. You can also use calcium supplements, such as egg shell powder or calcium carbonate, which appear to be two of the most easily used calcium sources by your body.

Phosphorus (phosphate)

Phosphorus is the second most abundant mineral in your body next to calcium.

Both calcium and phosphorus work together to help form strong bones and teeth, and about 85% of your body's phosphorus can be found there. Phosphorus can also be seen in your cells and tissues all over your body. Phosphorus helps filter out waste in your kidneys and helps with energy storage and usage. Phosphorus is also needed for growing, maintaining and repairing tissues and cells. Additionally, it is used in producing DNA and RNA.

Although you could potentially become deficient in phosphorus, it is highly unlikely that you would, and most people get enough phosphorus in their diet without even having to think about it at all. In fact, many people get too much phosphorus and not enough calcium, which could upset the calcium to phosphorus ratio we discussed earlier in the section on calcium. It may be a good idea to either try and reduce phosphorus, or increase calcium to help maintain about an equal balance of the two minerals.

Dairy is fairly high in phosphorus, but is also high in calcium as well, so they help balance each other out. Some foods that are high in phosphorus, but not in calcium, are many grains, nuts, seeds, and meat. If you have a diet high in those types of foods, you may want to supplement with extra calcium. Just eating more dairy products will add calcium into your diet, but dairy also has phosphorus in it as well. So adding dairy to an already phosphorus-rich diet would not necessarily balance things out. Unfortunately, it is easier to find foods high in phosphorus and low in calcium. It is not as easy to find foods high in calcium and low in phosphorus, which is why supplemental calcium may be helpful to some.

Magnesium

Magnesium is a mineral needed for the contraction and relaxation of your muscles, as well as helping more than 300 enzyme processes function correctly. Magnesium is also needed for the production and transport of energy, specifically oxidative phosphorylation and glycolysis, which help make the molecule ATP. ATP is basically the building block your body needs to create energy and keep your body running. In addition, magnesium helps in making new protein structures in your body, like muscle, skin, and internal organs.

Magnesium is an important mineral that plays a part in many critical functions in your body. Because of magnesium's crucial role in keeping your body running, it is a good idea to keep an eye on your magnesium intake to assure you do not fall too low. Magnesium is not found in high quantities in many foods, so getting the recommended amount of magnesium through food alone is difficult for many people. Sometimes it is easier to supplement if you feel you are low in magnesium.

The major reason why magnesium can be tough to get through food alone is because some of the highest foods in magnesium are either high-calorie foods like nuts, seeds and chocolate that may add too many calories, or fat, to your diet. And by the time you reached your goal of magnesium, you may not have enough room for other foods you want without going over your calorie or fat goals.

On the other hand, there are some lower calorie foods that have a high percentage of magnesium like spinach and Swiss chard, but you'd have to eat so much of those that it may not be appetizing or convenient just to get your goal of magnesium.

For example, almonds have some of the highest amounts of magnesium of any food. According to the RDA, the recommended intake of magnesium for a 31-50 year old man is 420 mg per day. In order to get that from almonds, you would need to eat 1.64 cups, which would be 902 calories, and 77 grams of fat. Depending on your calorie and fat goals, that can "crowd out" a significant portion of other options for your day.

Looking at the other option, spinach, which is another food with one of the highest amounts of magnesium, you would need to eat 17.7 cups of raw spinach to meet that 420 mg goal. (You could cook the spinach, but for the sake of measurement we'll use raw.) 17.7 cups of spinach is only 122 calories, but that's a lot of spinach. And it's doubtful that anyone could keep that up on a consistent basis.

Also keep in mind that foods like spinach and nuts contain substances like phytic acid that can block the absorption of minerals. With those sources, you may be absorbing less magnesium and other minerals, than they are reported to contain.

Basically, it's difficult to get enough magnesium by relying on one food alone. It's better to have a combined effect of eating relatively high magnesium foods. For example, let's say you had a dinner and dessert that included a large potato, one cup of Swiss chard, one cup of milk, and half a bar of dark chocolate. Combined, you'd have about 238 mg of magnesium, which is over half of that 420 mg goal, and would be a total of 544 calories. You can be creative with how you combine higher magnesium foods throughout your day to create recipes that you enjoy.

But remember that balance is key, and worrying about magnesium alone probably won't do you too much good. If you are at all concerned about your intake, you can enter your foods into an online nutritional tracker and see how you're doing. If you feel like you're low in magnesium, you can include different foods, or you could supplement, or maybe just be OK with a lower than RDA recommended value. It's your choice.

Manganese

Manganese is a mineral found in several foods, including nuts, legumes, seeds, tea, whole grains, shellfish, oatmeal, and leafy green vegetables. Manganese is considered an essential nutrient because the body requires it to function properly.

Some doctors use manganese as a medicine. Manganese can be used for prevention and treatment of "manganese deficiency," a condition in which the body doesn't have enough manganese. It is also used for weak bones (osteoporosis), anemia and symptoms of premenstrual syndrome.

Make sure to look out for manganese hidden in supplements and drugs. Certain supplements, including some that are commonly used for osteoarthritis, contain manganese. When using these products, it's important to follow label directions carefully. At amounts slightly higher than the recommended dose, these products provide more than the tolerable Upper Limit (UL) for adults, 11 mg of manganese per day. Consuming more than 11 mg per day of manganese could cause serious and harmful side effects.

But it would be difficult to get too much manganese in your diet by only eating whole foods, so supplements are mostly what you need to watch out for in regards to getting excessive manganese.

Zinc

Zinc is a mineral important for many functions in your body. Some of the most relevant to zinc are keeping your immune system strong, helping heal wounds, and assisting in creating new proteins and DNA.

Because zinc is used in creating new tissue, it is especially beneficial when you are growing as a child or when pregnant. Zinc is also helpful for athletes and bodybuilders because they are often breaking down muscle tissue and creating new muscle in its place.

Shellfish, especially oysters, are the best food sources of zinc, with red meat coming in second. Other foods, such as beans, nuts, and whole grains, also contain some zinc, but in significantly lower amounts, and some substances contained in those plant sources may partially block zinc's ability to be absorbed.

Generally, people tend to get enough zinc in their diet without even trying. That being said, if you have a high activity level, or lift weights regularly, then you may benefit from a higher zinc intake due to the increased need for tissue regeneration. Vegetarians or vegans may also need more zinc in their diet due to their avoidance of shellfish and red meat.

But too much zinc can be an issue as well, as excessive zinc can deplete the copper in your body, and create other issues. In addition, calcium can interfere with zinc's absorption, so if you're purposefully trying to eat foods with more zinc, or if you're supplementing with zinc, it's best to limit your calcium intake around the time you eat or supplement zinc. Again, the theme is balance.

Copper

Copper is a mineral component of key several enzymes required for a normal metabolism. While copper is an important element of your metabolism, it can also help to keep excessive iron out of your cells. If enough copper is not present in your cells, then iron can take the place of the spot normally reserved for copper. Once iron is in the spot where copper should be, then copper can't get in, so getting enough copper is important to make sure copper can occupy your cell before too much iron gets in copper's way.

Good food sources of copper are shellfish, organ meats, nuts, beans and chocolate. Many people get some copper just from their tap water because of the copper piping used to transport water.

The government did not have a recommended daily intake for copper until recently. And even now, the recommendations are a simplified form, as they only have an "adults" classification.

Iron

Iron is needed by virtually every cell in your body. It is responsible for helping in many processes. Two of the most important include helping your red blood cells carry oxygen to other cells, and being part of many important enzymes that help with cell functions.

Iron is found in a great variety of foods, mostly because iron is added to most grain based industrial or processed foods, such as bread and cereal. Some common non-processed foods with high concentrations of iron are red meats, shellfish, and beans.

Your body does need iron, but excessive iron can create accelerated oxidation, and therefore oxidative stress. If you've ever seen a rusty piece of iron, that's basically "oxidized" iron. Too much oxidation can also make your cells "rusty," and that "rust" can cause damage to your cells. This damage can accelerate aging and create a host of other potential issues.

As discussed above, one of the ways to prevent too much iron from getting into your cells is to make sure you are getting sufficient copper. Intentionally supplementing iron can be problematic for many people because excessive iron accumulation in cells can create damage.

It has been said that low iron can create anemia. Anemia is another way of saying you have a low amount of a substance called hemoglobin in your red blood cells. Many people will recommend increasing iron intake to help create more hemoglobin. This can help many people increase their hemoglobin number and alleviate symptoms of anemia. While increasing iron can be effective, it may not be the best option in all cases.

There are many reasons why your body would not produce enough hemoglobin, and a lack of iron is not always the reason. The potential issue with adding iron when you are not low in iron to begin with is that you may be pushing excessive iron into your tissues, creating free radicals, and causing damage to your cells. It is important to find out from your doctor if you do, in fact, have low levels of iron in your cells before you increase your iron intake. This is important to find out because there are a significant amount of options available to help with anemia outside of increased iron.

What makes this issue even more confusing is that your body will often produce extra hemoglobin when it has increased oxidative stress. So, even if you are not low in iron, adding iron may increase your oxidative stress, and therefore increase your hemoglobin, which may help with anemia. Although that may work to alleviate symptoms of anemia, there could be much less stressful and less damaging ways of solving the problem of anemia than increasing iron intake. Some of the potential alternative options are increased protein intake, and checking your thyroid function. However, if in fact you have low iron and you are anemic, then increasing iron may be an appropriate short term solution until you have restored normal iron levels.

Because iron can build up in your tissues over a lifetime and cause damage, it can be important to just get enough iron, and no more. If you find that you are high in iron, it is advisable to reduce your iron intake for enough time to normalize your iron stores. It is rarely a good idea to increase your iron levels purposefully without medical reason.

If you are purposefully attempting to reduce your iron intake, it can be difficult because iron is found almost everywhere, especially because industrial grain-based foods are likely to have iron added to them. However, taking calcium with iron-rich foods can help to block iron's absorption. Coffee can have similar blocking effects on some forms of iron. It can also be helpful to note that vitamin C taken with iron will increase iron's absorption potential. So avoiding the combination of vitamin C and iron can be helpful for limiting excessive iron intake.

Selenium

Selenium is an important mineral for your body. It is needed for a wide variety of functions, some of the most important being thyroid hormone metabolism, ability to protect against oxidative stress damage and infection, as well as helping to create new DNA.

Getting enough selenium can be a bit of a challenge just because it's not found in high concentrations within many foods. The highest concentration of selenium is in Brazil nuts, and even eating two Brazil nuts a day has been shown to help increase selenium levels in humans. Other nuts also have selenium, but nowhere near what Brazil nuts contain. Selenium can also be found in high concentrations in shellfish and seafood such as tuna. In smaller amounts, selenium can also be found in whole wheat products, eggs, milk, and muscle meat such as beef, lamb and poultry.

Salt

Salt is an integral mineral in our bodies. We need salt to help with retaining fluid. Salt can also help take excess water from inside our tissues and move it into our blood instead. Salt is also an electrolyte, which can help carry electrical impulses throughout our bodies, and that assists with muscle contraction and nerves firing. Getting enough salt can also help you retain more magnesium and potassium in your cells.

Determining how much salt to get in your diet is a tricky matter. Even the Center for Disease Control has admitted they do not know how much salt is too much, or how much is too little. Although they do concede that there are obvious health issues that can occur if you do not get enough salt, it is still difficult to determine how much salt is too much.

It appears that not getting enough salt is more of an issue than getting too much. Because of this, it is probably safe to say you can determine your own salt intake by deciding if something tastes too salty or not salty enough. Basically, just salt to taste and you should be fine. Worrying about reducing your salt intake is most likely not worth the effort, and could be more harmful than helpful, unless you have a medical reason to do so.

Potassium

Just like salt, potassium is also an electrolyte and is important for your body to work correctly. Potassium is needed for proper heart function, and helps with other muscle contractions as well, specifically smooth muscles like the muscles found in your digestive tract.

It can be important to balance your salt intake with potassium, meaning it may be a good idea to increase your potassium intake to closely match your salt intake. Some evidence suggests that the potential negative effects of salt only come into play when people don't get enough potassium along with the salt.

Potassium can be found in many foods, with some of the highest concentrations of potassium in orange juice, bananas, dried apricots, potatoes, and white beans. Potassium can also be found in significant quantities in most animal meats, fish and milk.

Although potassium is easily found in many foods, the RDA has some pretty steep requirements for potassium and getting the recommended amounts can be difficult. It may be more important to balance your salt to potassium intake rather than try to hit any specific number.

Iodine

Iodine is an essential element in thyroid hormones, specifically T3 and T4. In addition, iodine can help with immune and other biochemical reactions, such as protein synthesis and enzymatic activity.

Getting enough iodine is important, and a lack of iodine can cause your thyroid gland to swell up into a "goiter." However, getting too much iodine can also cause similar negative symptoms. It is best to get just enough iodine, and not intentionally increase your levels unless you have medical reason to do so. If you do require additional iodine for some reason, it may be good to note that taking extra selenium with iodine may be able to protect against excess iodine toxicity. It is also worth noting that most natural sources of iodine also contain selenium.

Some of the highest concentrated food sources of iodine include seaweed, shellfish, and other seafood. Potatoes also include high levels of iodine. Iodine is contained in smaller amounts in foods such as milk and eggs. Most "table salt" has iodine added to it as well.

That's it for the vitamins and minerals you should care most about. It's a lot to keep track of, so how could you possibly put together a plan that included all the vitamins and minerals you need without spending hours meal planning, cooking, and thinking about food every second of every day?

Well, the good news is that The First Diet makes this easy. And in the next chapter we are finally going to explore exactly what The First Diet is and why it works.

Chapter 12

THE FIRST DIET REVEALED

I hope you didn't skip right to this chapter. I mean, I understand if you jumped ahead, because this is where we'll really start getting into the details of The First Diet, but if you did fast forward—please do yourself a favor and go back to read the previous chapters. If you didn't, you won't fully appreciate and understand the beauty of The First Diet. If, however, you've made it this far, congratulations! You now know more about nutrition than most people ever will. Understanding nutrition and putting it into action are two different things, however, so let's start diving into The First Diet.

I want you to understand why this works. Not only so you can correctly use The First Diet for your benefit, but because understanding the fundamentals behind The First Diet has many benefits even beyond this diet. If you understand what The First Diet is, and also why it works, then you will be prepared to be flexible and creative in situations you may not expect. It's these unexpected situations or scenarios where you can't make something fit exactly into The First Diet that will cause the most failures, but it doesn't have to be that way, things don't have to fit perfectly all the time, rules are meant to be bent, and sometimes broken, but you need to understand the rules in order to bend and break them. If you simply read what foods, recipes, and quantities are included in a diet, then I would contend that you don't understand the diet fully, and you will be destined to fail.

I want you to succeed, and that is exactly why we went over key fundamentals of nutrition, such as how protein, carbohydrates, and fats react in your body. We went over vitamins and minerals, and we even covered psychological aspects and how stress can influence your blood sugar. I hope you understand how important this is. So if you've made it this far into The First Diet, I commend you, thank you for pushing through, I know it's not easy and I appreciate your effort.

Now it's time to put everything together. Let's go through what we've learned so far.

- Sugar is not the evil substance it's made out to be by the media. Sugar is efficient energy for your body, and sugar is brain food.
- Saturated fat is the most stable fat, and monounsaturated is the second most stable fat. Because of the stability of these fats, they are less likely to oxidize in your body and they are more likely to keep your body stable when you eat them. Polyunsaturated fats like omega-6 and omega-3 are unstable in comparison, and are much more likely to oxidize and create free radical damage to the cells and mitochondria inside your body.
- Protein is needed for your body to heal and repair. Diversifying your protein is a smart strategy, especially eating "nose to tail," which means including connective tissues and organs, as well as muscle meat. Connective tissues contain the amino acid glycine, whereas muscle meats like steak and chicken breast do not. And organs, especially liver, are packed with vitamins and minerals.
- Stress can originate in your mind from upsetting thoughts, or stress can originate in your body from nutritional deficiencies, such as not eating enough carbohydrates or calories. Stress speeds up the aging process in your body, and can destroy your health. You will likely never be able to get rid of all stress, and some stress is good, but stress should be minimized as much as practically possible.
- Vitamins and minerals are essential to your health. Getting a wide variety and doing your best to hit the RDA values in all the categories can have a positive impact on your health.

All right, so now we know all of this, but what do we do next? I mean, sure, you get it, sugar, saturated fat, diversified protein, minimize stress, and get your vitamins and minerals. But that's not very specific. And getting specific can sound difficult and complicated.

The good news is that it seems complex mostly because all the information we have about diet and nutrition today is all reverse-engineered based on what our bodies need to survive and thrive. At some point in the past all of this stuff must have just been baked into our environment. It must have just been available for us to access within our grasp, without even thinking about nutrition.

All these nutritional requirements didn't come from thin air; they weren't invented by science or research. These requirements were created by nature, inside of nature. Deep within where we were born. Orca whales were born in the sea, deer are born in the forest, alligators are born in the swamp, and all of the foods they need to thrive are in those places. Humans were born in the tropics, and that's where our food is. The food we need to thrive is the same food where we began, the same place we grew our big brains, the same place our first human fossils were found 200,000 years ago in East Africa.

With this knowledge in mind, we just need to see what was living in tropical East Africa 200,000 years ago, and what tends to grow there now. What food sources thrive in 98.6 degree weather?

Of course, we don't really know exactly what was growing in East Africa 200,000 years ago. Plants have changed, new species of plants have been added, animals have migrated, and some may have gone extinct. The weather was surely different as well. We can look back at trends to see what happened to our climate during that time and what was likely there. Let's make some educated guesses right now. I say guesses because there is no way to know for certain, but we can be fairly sure about some basic things.

Where our first human ancestors' fossils were found was likely a tropical or tropical-savanna environment. The basic structure of plants has not changed drastically in 200,000 years. One of the things that has not changed is in Africa is the fruit trees and palm trees. Fruit trees obviously produce fruit, but palm trees are a little more diverse. Palm trees can produce a variety of products, from coconuts, to sugar dates, to palm oil. The palm trees indigenous to tropical Africa did not include the coconut, as that was originally from Asia. These plants may have changed slightly, but not much in the way of their basic ability to produce sugar from fruit and dates, and saturated and monounsaturated fat from red palm oil.

There are many types of fruit indigenous to Africa. Most of them you have probably never heard of, as they are not commercially sold, but many have been analyzed for their nutritional content, and they are almost identically sweet to what we find in our modern fruit today. According to the book *Lost Crops of Africa,* there are over 1,000 different species of wild fruit in Africa from 85 botanical families. The book admits this assessment is likely incomplete and there are conceivably even more. Some of these fruits that you can find today are the junglesop, African custard apple, soursop, canistel, masuku fruit, gingerbread plum, pedalai, jaboticaba, bacupari, and the abiu. Nutritional analysis shows that the calories of these types of wild tropical fruits are almost completely made of sugar[10].

In the tropical environment of Africa, there were likely also many varieties of tubers, or potatoes as we know them today[11]. These ranged from larger yams to smaller egg-like tubers. There were also a great deal of above-ground green leafy plants, such as kale, the leaves of pumpkin-like-gourds, and spinach-like tropical plants such as Basella alba[11].

There is also evidence that humans were eating oysters at least 164,000 years ago in a cave in Africa[12]. And there is a good chance that humans were eating shellfish well before that time. Africa has a wide variety of saltwater and freshwater shellfish, from oysters to clams to mussels.

It is promising that ostriches were also roaming about. These ostriches may have been food sources to humans 200,000 years ago—both the ostriches themselves, and their eggs. At one of the oldest found human sites in Ethiopia, called "Omo 71", there were remains found of hippopotamuses, elephants, pigs, giraffes and fish[13]. This is likely where our tropical African ancestors got their protein.

So what do we have so far? Let's recap.

Our ancient tropical African ancestors likely ate:

- Root vegetables, like potatoes and yams
- Leafy greens, like kale and spinach
- Fruit, all sorts
- Sugar dates, from date palm trees
- Red palm oil, from oil palm trees
- Eggs, from ostriches or other birds
- Shellfish, like mussels and oysters

- Animals, like giraffes, elephants, pigs, and fish (nose to tail, connective tissues and organs)

Of course, The First Diet is not advocating that you now move to the tropics, grow palm trees in your backyard and eat giraffe steaks for dinner. That would be crazy. And difficult.

But we can translate those foods listed above into modern equivalents that have similar nutritional values, and which are likely available right now in your local grocery store. You can probably already see that some are easy to convert to modern foods, and others may be a little tougher. Let's give it a shot right now.

Root vegetables

You can find root vegetables like potatoes and yams at your local store. There is not nearly the same variety as you may be able to find all across Africa, but there are a decent amount of potato varieties at most supermarkets: russet potatoes, Yukon gold potatoes, red potatoes, sweet potatoes and yams, just to name a few. All of those potatoes are similar in nutritional content, and likely flavor, as you would have found in Africa 200,000 years ago.

Leafy greens

Leafy greens are easy to find at most supermarkets. They won't be the exact same variety as what is found in Africa, but they will be close. Kale and spinach are two easy greens to find in most modern stores, and they appear to match up very closely to what was found in Africa 200,000 years ago.

However, there is one key difference between the vegetables we have today and what is found in Africa. There is much more calcium in African vegetables according to Professor Abukutsa Mary Oyiela Onyango, a Professor of Horticulture at the Department of Horticulture, Jomo Kenyatta University of Agriculture and Technology. In one of her papers entitled, "African Indigenous Vegetables In Kenya," it states that just an average of 100 grams of fresh vegetables in Kenya contain levels of calcium that would provide 100% of your daily requirements. Kenya is right next to Ethiopia on the map, and remember that our first human fossils were discovered in Ethiopia.

100 grams of fresh vegetables is about ¾ of a cup. And while 100 grams of fresh vegetables in East Africa could provide 100% of your daily need for calcium, today the same amount of modern kale (one of the highest calcium vegetables you can find in supermarket grocery stores) would only provide approximately 135mg. That's falling short at only 14% of your RDA value for calcium. You would need almost 1,000 grams of modern kale to meet your daily calcium needs. In case you're wondering, 1,000 grams is about 15 cups of kale, that's a lot.

It's likely that our modern plants are lacking in magnesium as well. On the magnesium front, spinach is better than kale, but still low. 100 grams of raw spinach contains 70mg of magnesium. That's only 20% of your daily requirements. But remember how we mentioned our tropical African ancestors likely ate the leaves of pumpkins and other squashes? It's an educated guess that they didn't only eat the leaves; they also ate the entire squash and the seeds as well. 100 grams of squash seeds contains 534mg of magnesium, which is 134% of your recommended daily magnesium requirement. However, squash seeds include a significant amount of polyunsaturated fats, and 100 grams of seeds is about a cup. That's a lot of seeds to eat, just to reach your magnesium goals.

But don't worry, there are ways we can increase our calcium and magnesium intake without resorting to eating 15 cups of spinach, kale and pumpkin seeds. We'll talk about that a little later, but for now, it's important to realize that the calcium and magnesium levels of our plants today are likely lower than they were 200,000 years ago.

Fruit

Next is fruit, and luckily fruit is easy to find. All you need to do is walk into your local grocery store, and the produce aisle should be bustling with all sorts of different fruits: apples, bananas, grapes, mangoes, oranges, and more. The fruits found today are luckily still similar to what we had 200,000 years ago, at least in terms of sugar content.

Our fruit selection in modern society is robust. One catch is that many fruits are harvested early, and fruit is often put into stores much before they're ripe. This can lower some of the vitamins and minerals in modern fruit, and potentially make them a little less sweet than they should be in nature. But, these are small details and we're lucky to have access to as many fruits as we do today—pretty much no matter where you live.

Sugar

We know sugar is not hard to find, it seems like it's everywhere. That's a good thing. Our tropical African ancestors did not eat refined sugar, but they did have access to some type of sugar palm tree. The origin of these types of trees is not known due to their long cultivation, but they grow well in the Sahel region of Africa, which runs right next to Ethiopia. Approximately 200,000 years ago there was likely some type of date palm tree growing and available to our tropical African ancestors. Dates are essentially concentrated sugar; they are even shriveled up and almost dried out. Very close in composition to refined sugar.

Refined white sugar is often made from a plant called sugarcane. Sugarcane did not originate in tropical Africa, but sugarcane grows well in East Africa today, and sugarcane is a vital part of the economic growth of East Africa. Sugarcane is a tropical plant and also thrives in other tropical regions like Hawaii. Brazil is the leader in sugarcane production.

Refined white sugar is exactly what we talked about in the sugar chapter of this book. It is half glucose and half fructose. We already went over the benefits of sugar, but we didn't really touch on the negatives. White refined sugar, is not bad on its own, but it is devoid of any vitamins or minerals. It is simply sugar, and that's it. This is similar to white rice, or white flour, or any refined food. Many healthy people eat diets that include white rice and white flour as staples in their diet.

The problem comes when you eat a significant amount of your calories from foods that don't have much vitamins and minerals. These refined foods have calories that support your metabolism and your metabolism uses vitamins and minerals to function correctly. If your metabolism keeps running on refined fuel that is low in vitamins and minerals, your body will keep functioning, but eventually you'll start to run out of those vitamins and minerals. When you get deficiencies in vitamins and minerals, then your health can begin to falter.

Sugar (which is half glucose, and half fructose), tends to speed up your metabolism more than starch (which is almost completely glucose, and no fructose)—we covered the reasons why in a previous chapter. Because sugar speeds up your metabolism, it can also burn through vitamins and minerals faster. That means a diet that includes significant amounts of sugar should also be a diet that includes significant quantities of vitamins and minerals to support an increased metabolism. Unrefined sources of sugar that have more vitamins and minerals can be a better choice.

So, white sugar can be an absolutely healthy addition to your diet, but you must be mindful to also get enough vitamins and minerals along with that sugar. Because of this increased need for vitamins and minerals, it is best to eat sugar in as natural of a state as possible. This can be from juice or from the whole fruit itself. If your diet is nutrient-dense, then some extra white refined sugar should not hurt you at all under normal circumstances.

Palm Oil

There is no real need to purchase palm oil specifically at your grocery store. It is more important to understand what palm oil is made of so you can replicate the fats that found in palm oil. Palm oil is about half saturated fat and half monounsaturated fat, with a tiny bit of polyunsaturated fat in there as well. This really just means those fats are stable, as we talked about earlier in the chapter on fats.

You can easily replicate this idea by cooking with coconut oil, olive oil, and butter. Coconut oil is mostly saturated fat, olive oil is mostly monounsaturated fat, and butter is a mix of the two. Using these three stable fat sources will provide you with something similar to what is found in palm oil. You will get saturated, monounsaturated and a tiny bit of polyunsaturated fats. There are other sources of oil you can use as well; just check to see if they are mostly monounsaturated or saturated fat, and avoid the ones that have a significant amount of polyunsaturated fat.

If you're not sure if your oil is mostly monounsaturated or saturated, then you can do the refrigerator test. Just stick your oil in the refrigerator overnight, and if it's solid when you wake up, it's mostly stable fats. If it's still liquid in the fridge, it likely has a significant amount of polyunsaturated fats.

Eggs

Our tropical African ancestors probably ate whatever eggs they could find, such as ostrich eggs. Today, we can replicate that idea by using chicken eggs. Chicken eggs have a great deal of vitamins and minerals, especially in the egg yolks. To maximize the nutrition you receive from eggs, it is best to get them from pasture raised sources. Pasture raising chickens allows them to eat an ideal diet of bugs, seeds, and other forage plants. This gives the eggs more nutritional value and shifts the fats to be more stable.

If chickens are not pasture raised, they are often given soy feed, which has less nutrition and less stable fat. You can easily see this by cracking open two eggs, one pasture raised, and one from a factory-farm. The pasture raised yolk will be more firm and stable, it will stand up strong, and the color will be a dark orange. The factory-farmed egg yolk will be flimsy, break easily, not stand up tall, and the color will be a light yellow. Even factory-farm eggs contain a great deal of nutrition, but pasture-raised eggs contain even more.

Shellfish

Fresh shellfish is the best nutritional choice, and the best tasting. Fresh shellfish can be hard to find if you don't live by the coast, but even canned shellfish like oysters can be extremely high in nutrition.

If you find canned shellfish, make sure to check the type of oil they are preserved in. Oftentimes the oil will be high in polyunsaturated fat. If all you can find is shellfish floating in polyunsaturated fat oil, then just drain the fat and pat the shellfish dry with paper towels if you would like to remove the polyunsaturated oil.

Fish

Warm water fish, or "whitefish", are the best, as they contain low levels of polyunsaturated fat and low levels of fat in general. Some examples of warm water, or whitefish, are cod, halibut, rockfish, pollock, catfish, grouper, haddock, and sole. Tuna also works well, as it's a warm water fish and contains relatively low levels of fat.

Animals

As you know, finding animal products to eat is not difficult to do in our modern world. However, picking the animals that are most like what we encountered 200,000 years ago in tropical Africa is what we will highlight here. The good news is, that's pretty easy.

All we need to do is focus on ruminant animals, the ones with the four stomachs that convert polyunsaturated fats into saturated fats. The easiest ruminant animals to find in a modern grocery store are beef and lamb. Beef and lamb have a good mix of saturated and monounsaturated fats, and a little bit of polyunsaturated as well.

Chicken is a good option, but unless the chickens are pasture raised, they are likely high in polyunsaturated fats due to the farm feed. If you want to eat chicken regularly and avoid high levels of polyunsaturated fats, then focus on the less fatty cuts, like chicken breast.

Pigs are also the same as chickens in this respect. Factory-farm raised pigs are fed diets high in polyunsaturated fat. As a result, these pigs have high levels of polyunsaturated fat in their tissues, which then makes it into your tissues when you eat them. So when eating pork, it is best to focus on the less fatty cuts, or find pasture-raised pigs.

Making sure to eat "nose to tail" is also important in The First Diet, and our tropical African ancestors almost certainly ate this way as well. But it's not realistic to go get a whole animal and literally eat it from nose to tail. However, what you can do in our modern world to replicate that idea is to eat gelatin. Gelatin is primarily made from hooves, snouts, and skin.

You can make your own gelatin-rich bone broth from the feet of animals. Chicken feet work well for making low-fat, high-gelatin broths. As we discussed earlier, gelatin is the substance that helps round out our amino acid profile, and gelatin is the protein in animal skin and connective tissues.

A big part of eating "nose to tail" is including organ meats in your diet. The most nutrient rich organ is liver. Liver is considered a delicacy in many cultures, and there are a great deal of fancy dishes made from liver, such as foie gras and pâté. However, many find liver repulsive. If you do not enjoy liver, but still want to include it in your diet, there are companies that make liver pills from dried liver. That way you can get the nutritional benefits of liver without having to actually eat and taste it.

If you go the liver pill route, make sure to get the liver pills that still leave the fat inside. Some companies "defat" the liver and that takes out the vitamin A. Liver is the richest source of vitamin A you can get, and you don't want to leave the vitamin A out.

Translation summary:

We started with a list of foods that our tropical African ancestors ate, and then we translated those original foods to their modern food equivalents.

Here's a quick summary of the modern First Diet foods you can find in your local grocery store:

Potatoes—all kinds, shapes and sizes, white potatoes, sweet potatoes, yams and more. (Bonus: squashes like butternut squash and pumpkin fit in here too.)

Leafy greens—kale, spinach and anything that looks like them.

Fruit—all kinds, the sweeter the better.

Sugar—preferably natural sources like honey, but refined sugar is great too in moderation.

Oil/fat—saturated and monounsaturated fats are best, such as coconut oil, olive oil, and butter.

Eggs—chicken eggs are the easiest to find. Pastured chickens make the most nutrient dense eggs.

Shellfish—oysters, mussels and clams have the most nutrients. Fresh is best, but canned works too.

Fish—cod, halibut, rockfish, pollock, catfish, grouper, haddock, sole, tuna, etc. Warm water fish or whitefish with low polyunsaturated fat content are best.

Animals—ruminant animals like cows are ideal because, even if they are factory-farmed, they have stable saturated and monounsaturated fats. Pasture raised chickens and pigs are good sources as well. Liver is the most important organ meat to include in The First Diet due to its extremely dense nutrient value. Connective tissues, or gelatin, help round out your amino acid profile and make it easier to eat "nose-to-tail".

One last issue we must cover is the potential calcium and magnesium deficiency we mentioned previously. While it is possible to get your magnesium from sources like seeds and nuts, you'd have to eat an uncomfortable amount every day to get your recommended daily value of magnesium. In addition, nuts and seeds contain a significant amount of polyunsaturated fat.

In order to get your recommended daily value of calcium, you would also have to eat an agonizing amount of leafy green vegetables a day. This is technically possible, but it would not lead to a sustainable or pleasurable diet.

Because our plants tend to be giving us less calcium and magnesium than they once were, nature may have responded to that reality by giving humans a gift. That gift was a small genetic mutation known as "lactase persistence". Lactase persistence is the continued activity of an enzyme called "lactase" into adulthood.

Before lactase persistence developed in humans, we would stop being able to break down the lactose in our mother's milk after we stopped breastfeeding. Basically, once we weren't relying on our mother's milk any longer, we would lose the ability to digest milk. Around 7,500 years ago we suddenly became able to digest lactose for our entire human lives. However, there are still populations of humans who do not have lactase persistence, and are unable to process lactose. This condition is known as "lactose intolerance".

But those who can digest milk were given the benefit of easy access to calcium and magnesium. Ruminant animals like cows and goats eat plants all day long. They are easily munching up the 15 cups of leafy greens you would need to consume each day, and converting it into concentrated calcium and magnesium for us—along with many extra bonus nutrients. Just four cups of 2% cow's milk gives you 117% of your daily value of calcium, and gets you to 26% of your daily magnesium needs. As you can observe, milk is more weighted toward calcium than magnesium, but seeing as magnesium is not easy to get in nature, this is a big step in the right direction.

Of course, you do not need to drink four cups of milk every day, but even drinking two 8 ounce glasses would get you to 58% of your calcium needs, and 14% of your magnesium needs. Easy to do, and that's a compelling boost of nutrients.

In addition, milk contains a significant amount of protein, which can help your liver function and assist with muscle building and repair. Another positive to milk is that cows convert the polyunsaturated fats found in the plants they eat into stable saturated fats. If you can tolerate milk, it can be a positive way to bump up your protein, calcium and magnesium intake with very little added polyunsaturated fats. Milk is essentially concentrated plant power in liquid form with low polyunsaturated fat and lots of vitamins and minerals.

Another additional, and optional, First Diet food is coffee. Coffee originated in Ethiopia, close to where our first human remains were found[1]. The first documented discovery of coffee was made in the 9th century by a goat herder. The goat herder's name was Kaldi, and he discovered that his goats became excited after eating the beans from a coffee plant. Although interesting, this story is said to be apocryphal, meaning more myth than truth. The truth may be that coffee was discovered, and consumed, far before the 9th century.

Of course, we shouldn't just eat a food because something existed in nature at the location and time of where we evolved as a species. We should take the information about the fact that the food originated from the area of our origin and cross reference it with science—as we have been doing this whole book. Coffee is no different, and the studies on coffee indicate that it is potentially a powerfully healthy substance. However, as caffeine is a drug, some people respond to it favorably and others do not enjoy the effects of caffeine. For that fact, coffee is optional on The First Diet. That being said, let's talk about some of the benefits of coffee.

Coffee has been shown to:

- Increase the metabolisms of humans and help burn fat[2]
- Protect liver function and help keep human livers healthy[3,4]
- Help reduce the risk of Parkinson's Disease[5]
- Protect against developing Diabetes type 2[6]

And that's just some of the more important findings. Coffee consumption has many documented health benefits, and if you enjoy coffee it can be a useful addition to The First Diet. Keep in mind that because coffee can speed up your metabolism, and an increased metabolism requires more glucose to run, it can be a good idea to drink coffee with some sugar, or some carbohydrates on the side to keep your blood sugar regulated.

One more bonus item in The First Diet is chocolate. Chocolate did not originate in Africa. Instead, chocolate came from the tropical region of South America. Chocolate will only grow in hot climates that are within 20 degrees of the equator. And although chocolate did not emerge from Africa, it thrives there. Today, nearly 70% of all chocolate is grown in Africa.

Like coffee, chocolate is completely optional on The First Diet. Chocolate is primarily saturated fat and sugar, which are two fundamental elements in The First Diet, so chocolate fits in under these guidelines. But chocolate is not just sugar and saturated fat.

Chocolate has some unique qualities, and chocolate has been shown to:

- Have unusually high levels of antioxidants[7]
- Help increase brain function[8]
- Help prevent fat gain[9]

Now, on the last point—regarding the fact that chocolate may help prevent fat gain—it is important to note that any food someone overeats can contribute to fat gain. However, researchers in Spain studied the diets of 1,458 teenagers, and the results showed that the teens who ate the most chocolate had the least body fat. Less body fat overall, and less fat in their middle region.

Chapter 13

PUTTING IT ALL TOGETHER

We now have a list of foods we have translated from our tropical African ancestors into our modern times. We realize that sugar, especially from fruits, can be beneficial. We understand that stable fats like saturated and monounsaturated fats are best for our 98.6 degree bodies, and that polyunsaturated fats don't do so well at our body temperatures, or inside of our bodies. In addition, we recognize that eating nose-to-tail is important to get enough protein from muscle meats as well as connective tissues, and organ meats like liver are powerfully nutrient dense.

It's time to show you how all these foods can fit together to fulfil your daily carbohydrate, protein and fat needs, as well as your vitamin and mineral needs.

Just to recap, here's a list of the foods we talked about again:

- Root vegetables (potatoes, carrots, onions, etc.)
- Leafy greens
- Fruit
- Sugar
- Coconut oil
- Olive oil
- Eggs
- Shellfish
- Fish
- Animals, nose-to-tail (bone broths, gelatin, and liver)
- Milk (optional but encouraged)

- Chocolate (optional)
- Coffee (optional)

And for purposes of illustration, here's what a diet with these foods looks like in terms of their vitamin and mineral values when put together on even a very low calorie diet. This example is not recommended; it is purely to show that even with small amounts of these foods you can still reach extremely high levels of vitamins and minerals.

This example would not be recommended for two reasons. Reason one, this is too low of calories for almost anyone. Reason two, no thought has gone into the flavors of this diet illustration, it would likely be a gross combination of foods without some thought about specific recipes. Again, the following example is purely given so you can see how these foods, with even low calories, pack a nutritional punch.

Example diet: (Do not try this at home. This is for illustration of nutrient value only.)

- Two cups of 2% milk
- Two cups of orange juice
- One medium banana
- Two large eggs
- One ounce of beef liver
- One mango
- One cup of kale
- One cup of spinach
- One small oyster
- One cup of gelatin-rich bone broth
- One medium baked white potato

All of this comes to only 1,341 calories. Even with this small of a calorie count, let's take a look at what this gives us in terms of vitamins and minerals.

- Vitamin B1 = 91%
- Vitamin B12 = 1,063%
- Vitamin B2 = 267%
- Vitamin B3 = 108%
- Vitamin B5 = 166%
- Vitamin B6 = 288%
- Folate = 193%
- Vitamin A = 1,560%
- Vitamin C = 441%
- Vitamin E = 71%
- Vitamin D = 170%
- Vitamin K = 1,644%
- Calcium = 110%
- Copper = 537%
- Iron = 188%
- Magnesium = 103%
- Manganese = 156%
- Phosphorus = 182%
- Potassium = 110%
- Selenium = 169%
- Sodium = 62%
- Zinc = 121%

And that's not all. With these foods we had only 3.7 grams of polyunsaturated fat, and the rest were saturated and monounsaturated.

As you can see, we are a little low on two things here. Number one was vitamin E, and number two was sodium. In terms of vitamin E, you tend to need more vitamin E the more polyunsaturated fats you eat. Vitamin E is an antioxidant, and it helps combat against the potential damage polyunsaturated fats can cause when they oxidize. If you eat fewer polyunsaturated fats, you likely need less vitamin E. Vitamin E tends to be included in natural foods that have polyunsaturated fats as well. If you eat more natural polyunsaturated sources, you'll get more vitamin E, but you'll also need more vitamin E because you'll need to protect against lipid peroxidation. In this case, the lower vitamin E is not a concern because of the small polyunsaturated content.

In regards to sodium, we did run a little low at only 62% of our daily requirements. That's OK because we didn't calculate any added salt in our food log—and added salt would increase our sodium numbers. So we would probably get more salt in our day than showed up in our numbers. Because, generally speaking, when you cook something, you'll add salt to it, adding salt to taste should increase our sodium levels to 100% or possibly a little over, which is absolutely fine. As long as you keep a good potassium to sodium ratio, you should be OK with extra salt intake. In this case we got 5 grams of potassium, and only 1 gram of salt. We could bring that salt intake up by potentially 4 grams to match the potassium and be in balance. So there's lots of room to play with salt here.

For at least 3 months or so, I recommend entering every piece of food you eat, every day, into an online nutritional log. There are many out there, but ideally choose one that keeps track of not only calories, protein, carbohydrates and fat, but also vitamins and minerals. At the time I'm writing this book, cronometer.com is a good choice. Keeping track of your food intake can be tedious, boring, and frustrating, but it will give you something invaluable: Over time, you will get an intuition for what foods are made of. You'll be able to look at the foods you eat and know with x-ray vision how many calories something is, how much protein, carbohydrates and fat it has, and also have a good idea of the vitamins and minerals inside each food. You will never be perfect at it, but getting that intuition developed will allow you to effortlessly make better choices.

Back to our example above, at 1,341 calories, we were much too low on energy for most people to stay happy, healthy and strong. Sure, we covered almost every single vitamin and mineral category, and that's the beauty of the foods in The First Diet, but vitamins and minerals are not everything. You need enough energy in the form of calories as well. The great thing about this example is that you have so much more room for flexibility. Many people can eat at least 2,000 calories a day and not gain weight. So in this case, we have around 700 calories on top to play with. This is where you could potentially add in some refined sugar, or white rice, or pleasurable foods that don't necessarily add much value in terms of vitamins and minerals, because you already have that covered.

Regardless of the vitamins and minerals we got in our example, you probably will not want to eat a little bit of liver, a little oyster, and kale and spinach every single day. And you don't need to. It really matters more that you average out to around 100% on many vitamins and minerals, not that you need to get exactly 100% every single day. For most people it would make much more sense to eat one meal a week that contains seven shellfish, not just one shellfish every single day. And no, it doesn't have to be exactly seven shellfish, I'm just trying communicate that in many cases the average matters, not an every-single-day thing. Seven shellfish, one day a week, divided by seven days in a week, is an average of one shellfish a day.

But there are certain vitamins and minerals that can be better to eat every day as opposed to weekly. Water soluble vitamins don't stick around in your body as well as fat soluble vitamins. Water soluble vitamins end up in your toilet much faster than fat soluble vitamins, which tend to stick around in your fat. Maintaining a steady daily supply of the water soluble vitamins is a good idea. With the fat soluble vitamins, you can eat larger quantities less frequently and they will stay in your body longer.

The B vitamins are water soluble, which includes thiamin (B1), riboflavin (B2), niacin (B3), pantothenic acid (B5), pyridoxine (B6), biotin (B7), folate (B9), and cyanocobalamin (B12). In The First Diet, or anywhere else, liver is going to be your most concentrated source of B vitamins. It's for this reason that eating a little liver every day can be beneficial to keep your energy and B vitamin levels strong. B vitamins are known to give an energy boost, and many popular energy drinks contain B vitamins for that reason. Of course, it's not absolutely required to eat a little liver every day, but some people feel better doing that, and others do not. You'll have to experiment yourself.

I've tried eating seven ounces of liver once a week, and eating about one ounce a day. I find that eating one ounce a day works best for me. There are a few ways to make eating a little liver a day easier. One way is to cut up the liver beforehand and freeze it, then you can take little bite sized pieces out of the fridge each day and eat them. Or you can get liver powder and get your liver in pill form. I find that the dried liver powder pills work well to give me energy, but not as well as fresh liver.

But liver does not just contain B vitamins; liver also has the highest concentration of bioavailable vitamin A in nature. Vitamin A is fat soluble, so you can eat 4-6 ounces once a week or so and you would still be able to store the excess Vitamin A. For example, 6 ounces of liver gives you approximately 958% of your daily requirements for vitamin A. If you do that once a week, then you can divide 958% by 7 days in a week, and you'd get an average of 136% of your daily value of vitamin A. That works well for many people.

Vitamin C is the other water soluble vitamin, and vitamin C is highly concentrated in fruit and fruit juice. If you even just drink one cup of orange juice a day, you would get approximately 93% of your vitamin C requirements in that alone. Eating fruit and drinking fruit juice regularly is the easiest way to keep your vitamin C levels up.

The rest of the vitamins and minerals will stick around for much longer in your body than water soluble vitamins. So getting a weekly average of the rest of the vitamins and minerals is more important than trying to hit 100% every single day. It's likely that you'll do something more like the example before, where you eat 958% of your vitamin A in one day of the week, and that averages out to 136% a day.

Although calcium and magnesium are not water soluble, it is important to keep a steady daily stream of those going. That's for two reasons. Reason one is that magnesium is difficult to get 100% of your recommendation every day, so if you skip 3 days and then need to make up 300%, that will be difficult. Also, too much magnesium at one time can cause intestinal discomfort.

In addition, if your body does not have enough calcium in your blood during the day, it will start taking the calcium it needs from your bones. You want to keep your bones healthy and strong, so maintaining a steady supply of calcium each day can help prevent your body using your bones for the calcium it needs. This is why drinking milk can be helpful.

So now that we understand that we can get 100% or more of our daily requirements of vitamins and minerals on The First Diet, we need to talk about how much protein, carbohydrates and fat is ideal. Because it's not just about vitamins and minerals, it's also about calories and where you get those calories from. Before we cover the topic of calories, we need to talk about why people gain weight, and what happens when they try to lose it. Knowing this information can be helpful in understanding what goes on in your body when you are gaining and losing weight. When you really get this, then you are more likely to have success and less likely to fall for bad advice in the future. You'll be able to tell if a weight loss plan is healthy or not.

Chapter 14

WHY PEOPLE GAIN FAT

Y ou probably know this, but it needs to be said. You can gain fat on any diet. There are physical realities about how your body works that no diet can overcome completely. Yes, you can lose fat on The First Diet, and we will talk about that in the next chapter. But first, you need to understand why people gain fat. A foundation must be laid down to build on.

Eating more than your body uses can, and probably will, cause you to gain weight. Keep in mind that weight gain is not the same thing as fat gain. There are many ways to gain weight. For example, storing carbohydrates in your muscles will cause weight gain on the scale, but probably won't make you appear any fatter.

Increasing muscle will also cause you to gain weight, and will make you appear more muscular if you accumulate enough. You can also boost your weight with greater bone density, and stronger ligaments and tendons. There are many ways to gain weight by eating more that will not necessarily contribute to body fat. Having said that, it is still possible that eating too much of anything can result in fat gain.

Why can eating too much contribute to fat gain? Let's explore the possible ways that fat gain can happen.

Fat gain scenario 1. Eating too much fat

Let's say you have already eaten enough protein and carbohydrates to provide your body enough energy to run for the day; while leaving room in your diet for an extra 50 grams of fat. You could eat that 50 grams of fat and not gain any fat, because eating that amount would be enough to cover your body's energy needs for that day with the combined protein and carbohydrates you ate before.

So let's say you eat the 50 grams of fat. What happens? You don't gain anything, your body stays the same weight, and you don't gain any fat— you also don't lose any fat. But, let's pretend that you ate the 50 grams of fat, and then you ate another 40 grams of fat on top of that.

In this case, your body does not need any more energy for the day to operate, and therefore will not burn that extra 40 grams of fat. As we know, the fat you eat gets stored in your body. If your body needs energy, it will be metabolized, but in our scenario your body does not need this extra fat for fuel today, so it will be stored and not used.

At the end of the day, you will have an extra 40 grams of fat stored in your body, and you will be 40 grams fatter. If this trend keeps up, then that 40 grams will end up being 80 grams, and then 160 grams stored. Soon those extra stored fat grams can become one pound, two pounds, five pounds and more of stored fat on your body.

Fat gain scenario 2. Eating too many carbohydrates

Again, let's say you have eaten enough fat and protein to cover your body's energy needs for today, while leaving in room for an extra 150 grams of carbohydrates. You could eat that 150 grams of carbohydrates and not gain any fat, because eating those carbohydrates would give your body enough energy to run on for the day with the combined protein and fat you ate before.

Things get a bit trickier with carbohydrates on a technical level, but let's keep things simple here because technical information doesn't always end up directly applying to real life. And technicalities can sometimes cause you to "lose the forest from the trees."

So, on a practical level, what happens if you eat those 150 grams of carbohydrates? You wouldn't gain any weight, and you wouldn't lose any weight. Your body would stay just about the same. But let's pretend you ate the 150 grams of carbohydrates plus another 80 grams of carbohydrates. What happens then? One of two things.

Situation one: If your muscles can store more carbohydrates, then those extra 80 grams of carbohydrates you ate can end up being stored as glycogen in your muscles. That extra glycogen will not convert to fat. However, you will gain body weight in the form of stored carbohydrates. The good thing is that these stored carbohydrates in your muscles will make your muscles appear bigger and fuller. When professional body-builders are dieting to very low calories, they lose a lot of stored carbohydrates in their muscles. This loss of carbohydrates makes their muscles look smaller.

Bodybuilders don't want their muscles to look smaller, so shortly before they go on stage for their competitions, bodybuilders will eat a large quantity of carbohydrates. This huge amount of carbohydrates fills up their muscles and makes them look as big as possible. These extra carbohydrates will make the bodybuilders gain instant weight on the scale, and they look like they got more muscular too. But none of the weight gain is fat; otherwise they wouldn't do it, because they want to be as lean as possible for their competition. This can happen to you as well when your muscles get bigger from storing carbohydrates, just probably not quite as dramatically.

Situation two: If your muscles are full up on glycogen, then some of the extra 80 grams of carbohydrates will most likely be converted to fat through a process called "de novo lipogenesis." However, de novo lipogenesis rarely happens in humans.

The process of converting carbohydrates to fat wastes a lot of energy, so the full 80 grams of carbohydrates will not convert to the same amount of body fat. Two conditions need to be met in order for carbohydrates to turn into fat. Condition one is that your body is completely full up on carbohydrate storage and cannot take in anymore carbohydrates. Condition two is the carbohydrates must be chemically converted into fat, and that wastes at least 33% of the energy in the carbohydrates and creates heat instead.

Even if you were completely full up on carbohydrate storage in your body and the carbohydrates you ate could turn into fat—carbohydrates are 4 calories per gram, and fat is 9 calories per gram. So, 80 grams of carbohydrates would be equal to about 36 grams of fat. 33% of that 80 grams would be wasted. After the 33% deduction and 9 calorie conversion, 80 grams of carbohydrates could convert to 23 grams of fat. And that's only if there is no possible room left in your body for carbohydrate storage, and then after you were completely full, you ate an extra 80 grams of carbohydrates, which is about two cans of soda.

Carbohydrates transforming into fat is not the way most people gain fat, even if they are eating too many carbohydrates. Most people gain fat when they eat excessive carbohydrates because they are also eating a significant amount of fat in addition to the carbohydrates. Your body likes to burn carbohydrates first because carbohydrates are your body's preferred fuel choice. If you give your body enough carbohydrates to function on all day long, plus more, then your body will run on carbs all day long. That can be a good thing, but if you also eat fat along with that surplus of carbs, then you won't burn the same amount of fat you ate, and you will have extra fat on your body at the end of the day.

So if someone is overeating on carbohydrates, and then includes fat in the equation as well, then the fat they eat will be likely to stay on their bodies for much longer. If someone wants to overeat on carbohydrates, it is best to combine that with a low fat intake to minimize fat gain.

Keep in mind that exercise can use up carbohydrates in your muscles. When you exercise and use stored carbohydrates in your muscles, that leaves room for more carbohydrate stockpiles. If you have room in your muscles for more carbohydrate storage, there is little chance that any carbohydrates will turn into fat. Carbohydrates turning into fat in humans is rare, and is not a significant contributor to fat gain. The real problem is too many carbohydrates combined with too much fat.

Fat gain scenario 3. Eating too much protein

Let's pretend that you have eaten enough carbohydrates and fat to give your body enough energy to run for today, while leaving room for an extra 50 grams of protein. You could eat that 50 grams of protein and you shouldn't gain any fat because eating that protein would give your body just enough energy to run for today—with the combined carbohydrates and fat you ate before.

So, if you eat those 50 grams of protein, you shouldn't gain or lose any weight or fat. But let's pretend you ate the 50 grams of protein plus another 80 grams of protein. What happens then?

One of two things:

Situation one

If your body has been performing strength training exercises, or something similar, and can use the extra protein to create bigger body structures, like muscle, then that protein can be utilized to build tissue, and will not be used for fat generation. At the end of the day, you will gain weight, but it will be in the form of new muscle or new support-structures in your body and not necessarily fat.

Situation two

If your body has not been strength training, or something like it, and does not have any reason to use the excess protein, then that protein can be converted to carbohydrates, or it can linger around in your system a bit longer. If your body turns protein into carbohydrates, then we are back at "fat gain scenario 2. Eating too many carbohydrates" and the same rules apply—you can use the carbohydrate for refueling your muscles, or if your muscles are full, you can convert it to fat.

As you can probably tell, excess protein is less likely to convert to body fat because protein does not convert directly to fat. It would need to transform to carbohydrates first. You would also need your muscles to be "maxed out" on their glycogen storage capacity in order for fat to be created from protein that was converted to carbohydrate first.

This is probably why people believe that if you eat more protein, you will be less likely to gain fat. The truth is, while protein will not directly turn into fat, the excess protein you eat, and are unable to use, will still temporarily inhibit fat burning due to a few factors. One major factor why protein can slow down fat burning in the short term is just like carbohydrates—protein can increase insulin, and while insulin is raised, fat burning tends to decrease. This temporary inhibition of fat burning will leave you more likely to keep your stored fat longer, and the excess energy will "spill over" into tomorrow's energy needs, so you will require a bit less calories tomorrow because of the "spill over" of energy. If you eat the same amount tomorrow as you did today, you "spill over" again and that window where your fat burning is slowed down will accumulate over time, and lead to more fat gain in the long term.

Because the system your body uses to store fat is complicated, many people will try to use that complication to find ways to "trick the system," or at least make a convincing argument as to why they think they are tricking the system. However, any food you overeat, whether protein, carbohydrate, or fat, can lead to fat gain over time. Some types of foods are less likely to convert to fat in the moment, but over time they will catch up to you if you continue to overeat. You can't cheat the system, even if someone makes a convincing argument on paper.

One major point that needs to be made is that sometimes fat gain is a good thing. In some situations fat gain can be the healthier option.

Keep in mind that the more active you are, the more your muscles will use carbohydrates, and they will have more storage room. More storage room means you are less likely to make fat from carbohydrates. In addition, the more muscle you build, the more protein you can use, and the more carbohydrates you can store. Those both make fat storage less likely, and the more mass and body weight you have, the more food you can eat and not gain weight as well. In addition, bigger muscles also burn more fat, even at rest.

So, bigger muscles can store more carbohydrates, which makes it less likely for fat gain to happen, and bigger muscles burn more fat. Having big muscles makes you less likely to store fat, and more likely to burn fat. That's a good combination, and it's why strength training can be helpful in fat loss and preventing fat gain.

Every type of food (protein, carbohydrates, and fat) has its place. None of them are evil by themselves, and none directly lead to fat gain by themselves.

We've talked about how eating an excess of any type of food can lead to weight gain, so now let's talk about what happens if you try to "trick" your body into losing weight by cutting out an entire macronutrient type (protein, carbohydrates or fat).

Your body is smart, smarter than many diet professionals would give it credit for. People often think that if they cut out, or cut way down on an entire food classification (protein, carbohydrates, or fat) they can somehow end up with better health, or increased weight loss.

Protein, carbohydrates and fat are all important to health, and we'll explore below what happens when you cut one out.

Scenario 1. Cutting out carbohydrates

Technically speaking, your body can run without the addition of carbohydrates in your diet. It can do this because of your body's ability to turn protein into carbohydrates. Also, if your body is forced to, it can create something called ketones. If you're making a significant amount of ketones and using those for energy, people call that "going into ketosis." While your body can run on ketones, and ketones are technically an "efficient" source of energy, being in ketosis is the result of a stressed state of your body, and your body will do almost anything possible to get out of ketosis as quickly as possible.

It is difficult to stay in ketosis for long periods of time, and any significant amount of protein you eat while in ketosis will be most likely used to create carbohydrates, and those carbohydrates will "pop" you out of ketosis quickly. Because of this, the only way to stay in ketosis for any extended period of time is to almost exclusively eat fat and very little protein. That way there is nothing for your body to use to make carbohydrates with any longer.

Many people lower their carbs, or almost eliminate them, while still eating a large amount of protein and fat. They believe they are cutting out carbs, but what they fail to realize is that the protein they are eating is turning into carbs in their bodies. So you can either eat carbs, or your body will turn protein into carbs. Either way, you've got carbs in your system. Your body is smarter than that.

There are many potential problems with consistently relying on protein to make carbohydrates in your body. One of the main issues is if you're trying to get enough protein to repair your body, or recover from workouts, the protein you are eating is not getting used for muscle repair purposes. Most of the protein you're eating (if you're not eating enough carbohydrates) is being used to turn back into carbohydrates, and essentially is making the protein you're eating not useful in the way that you had intended. Essentially, if you are eating protein and no carbs, then your body will "steal" that protein and use it as a carbohydrate. A low carb, high protein diet may end up as a medium protein, medium carbohydrate diet after all the "stealing" has been done.

All of that "stealing" is stressful, too. Converting protein into carbohydrates relies greatly on stress hormones to operate. And long term elevation of stress hormones can have negative effects on your health, so if you have the option of converting protein into carbohydrates through stress, or just eating carbohydrates, which would you chose? Turn a pot roast into a potato with some stress juice, or just eat the potato?

Scenario 2. Cutting out fat

Your body needs fat to function. If it doesn't get enough fat from your diet, it can make fat on its own if it's forced to. Or it can make fat if you are eating a great deal of carbohydrates and you are not significantly active. However, fat generation from carbohydrates does not happen extremely often. Cutting back on fat to a degree can be helpful for some people, but going too low can be detrimental to your health as well. It is not advisable to go lower than 10% of your calories from fat. Many people function better in the 20-30% calories from fat range.

Why can cutting back on fat too much be harmful? There are many fat soluble vitamins that rely on fat for absorption. Also, having enough fat in your diet, and even fat on your body, seems to be linked to better hormonal environments and increased overall health. Many people notice a drop in mood if they eat too little fat as well.

Regardless of how little fat you eat, if you still "overeat" with protein and carbohydrates, you will be at risk of gaining body fat due to factors discussed earlier.

Scenario 3. Cutting out protein

How much protein you need in your diet is a highly debated topic, but one point that everyone seems to agree on is this: Although your body can technically run without carbohydrates, and your body can make its own fat, your body cannot make its own protein. This is probably why you've never seen any protein elimination diets.

While you can technically live in the short term without eating protein, you probably won't do too well long term without protein in your diet. Cutting out protein completely would be difficult. Almost every variation of a human diet has protein in it, whether that protein comes from a plant or an animal.

The more carbohydrates you eat, the less protein you technically would need, due to the fact that less protein would be converted to carbohydrates, and more protein could be used for what protein is best at. If you eat enough carbohydrates to cover your body's needs, then your body will not be forced to convert protein to carbohydrates. Therefore, you can retain more lean muscle mass and use the protein you eat for good use. It can be said that carbohydrates are a protein protective substance.

If you don't eat protein long enough, you will probably end up breaking down your own body tissues, like muscle, in order to get the protein you need for repairs. Eventually your muscle would run out, and bad things would happen. But again, it would be difficult to get no protein in your diet pretty much no matter what you eat.

So we've seen that cutting out, or way down on, any large classification of food is probably not a good idea, and it seems like you can't "out smart" your body by eliminating macronutrients.

Often the reason a diet that cuts out entire food classifications works is because it makes it harder to find foods that you like to eat. Basically, the end result is that you may lose weight due to "accidentally" eating less out of inconvenience. Or maybe you eat less because eating a ton of calories in chicken breast and broccoli is difficult to stomach.

Make no mistake: These diets often do not work because they are doing something special to your body. They are usually working by reducing calories, even if that's not what they tell you. But there's an elegant way to reduce calories and still let your body run as stress-free as possible by giving it the carbohydrates it needs to function, the protein it needs to build and repair, and the fat it needs for hormone and mood regulation. That will be covered in the next chapter.

Chapter 15

CARBOHYDRATES, PROTEIN, AND FAT

Now we know how your body tends to respond to overeating on carbohydrates, protein, and fat. We also know what happens if you cut out an entire category, and how that can lead to problems. So how do we keep our systems balanced and running strong? Part of the equation is vitamins and minerals, and you already know that The First Diet, even with low calories, can give you 100% or more of your daily values of vitamins and minerals. However, vitamins and minerals are not the whole picture, so let's move to carbohydrates, protein and fat. We're going to put these together in a way that keeps your body as stress-free as possible, while giving you the tools to lose weight, maintain weight, or gain weight.

We want to keep the structure of your energy systems solid by eating stable fats, we want to keep your metabolism strong by eating enough sugar, and we want to let your body heal and build by giving it enough protein. And yes, the quantities of each matter.

Carbohydrates

Let's start with carbohydrates. We must give your body the carbohydrates it needs to optimize your metabolism, reduce stress, hold on to muscle, and give you energy.

Most people can run on about 200 grams of carbohydrates and fulfill their basic metabolic requirements. Some people need more carbohydrates if they are active, or if they have large muscles that take up lots of energy—or if they naturally have a higher metabolism. 200 grams of carbohydrates is on the lower end, and you may want to experiment with higher numbers. 300 grams of carbohydrates can be a better starting place for those who do not want to lose weight, but we'll get into this a little later. It doesn't absolutely matter if you get these carbohydrates from sugar (the sweet carbohydrate found in fruit, and other sweet-tasting plants), or starch (the not-so-sweet carbohydrate found in plants like potatoes).

However, remember that fruit sugar comes with more vitamins and minerals than white sugar, and sugar can increase your metabolism more than starch. Personally, I think it's a good idea to get at least 60% of your carbohydrates as sugar, and the rest from starch. Some people feel best with more sugar, and some people feel better with more starch. You'll have to find what works best for you.

Protein

For the majority of people, it is unnecessary to go over 100 grams of protein a day, unless you are extremely muscular, or highly active with intense exercise like sprinting, weight lifting, or other activities that tear down muscle fiber.

The lowest most people should go is 80 grams a day for overall metabolic function, and for retaining muscle. The highest should be somewhere around 1 gram of protein per pound of bodyweight. If you weigh 170 pounds, then 170 grams of protein is your maximum.

Fat

Fat is an important substance, and your body needs some fat to help absorb fat soluble vitamins, create hormones, and build structures in your body, like your brain. However, your body does not need a lot of fat to perform these functions. Because of that, it is best to keep your fat intake to about 55 grams a day if you are a woman and around 65 grams a day if you are a man.

The difference in fat intake is due to the fact that men burn fat faster than women, partly due to their higher muscle mass and testosterone[1]. Women do not burn fat at the same rate as men, so their fat intake should be slightly lower. This fat intake is not extremely low however, because at a 2,000 calorie diet, 65 grams of fat would still be about 30% of your total calories coming from fat.

If you feel the need to increase your calories, it may still be a good idea to hold fat at 55 or 65 grams, even if the 30% number goes down as your calories go up. The reason you may not want to increase your fat while you are increasing calories is that the fat you eat is the fat that is stored on your body, and as your calories go up, your ability to burn fat goes down. If you eat more fat, you'll be likely to store more fat. There is no reason to go very low in fat, but it is a good idea to watch your fat intake to make sure it does not go too high.

Total carbohydrate, protein and fat per day baseline summary

Carbohydrate (men and women):

- 200 grams minimum
- 300 grams average
- 300+ depending on activity and muscle mass

Protein (men and women):

- Minimum of 80 grams
- Maximum of 1 gram of your bodyweight (if you're trying to build muscle)
- Optimum 100 grams

Fat:

- Women 55 grams
- Men 65 grams

Regarding these numbers, I don't want to bring up fat loss or fat gain yet, but the nature of this conversation forces me to; because 200 grams of carbohydrates, 80 grams of protein and 65 grams of fat is a grand total of about 1,700 calories. 1,700 calories is not enough calories for most people to maintain their weight. In fact, most people will lose fat at this calorie range. For many people, it could be better to start at 300 carbohydrates and bring that calorie total to 2,100. Losing fat may be good for some, but others would rather not. If you find you are losing weight and do not want to, the easiest and most likely healthiest way to stop the fat loss is to keep your protein and fat the same and increase your carbohydrates. Basically you can use your carbohydrates as kind of a "brake pedal" for fat loss.

If you want to maintain your current weight, just keep increasing your carbohydrates until you find that you are not gaining or losing weight. Many people will tell you to "throw out the scale" because the numbers will drive you crazy. I say the exact opposite. I think you should weigh yourself at the same time every single day. Preferably, you should weigh yourself in the morning, right after you've gotten out of bed and done your "business". After you're done with your "business", step away from the toilet and onto your scale. Look at that number every single day.

That number on the scale will go up and down, and up and down. But over time you will see a pattern. Is it going up, up, down, up, up, up? If you're 10 pounds heavier than last month and the scale keeps trending up, then you're gaining weight. If the scale is going down, down, up, down, down, up, down, and you're 5 pounds lighter than last month, then you're losing weight. But if you don't look, every day, you will not see the pattern.

Do not be concerned with small fluctuations from day to day. Be more concerned with the overall trend. If you do this long enough, you will get an automatic intuition for where you are, and if you are gaining or losing. Just step on the scale every single day, and adjust your carbohydrates as needed.

You should also cross reference this with looking in the mirror every single day, and checking to see how your clothes fit each morning. These are probably things you do anyway, but it's important to cross reference the mirror and the fit of your clothes with your scale weight. You could be gaining weight on the scale, but you may not look any fatter, and your clothes may fit the same. In that case, the weight gain is likely due to the fact that you are gaining muscle, or storing more carbohydrates inside of your muscles. When you store more carbohydrates in your muscles, you will gain weight on the scale, but that weight will not be fat. Your muscles may look and feel bigger because they have more carbohydrates and water inside to use as fuel. As a bonus, this usually means you will feel more energetic, and be able to work out harder if you want to, because that extra weight is literally energy waiting to be used inside of your muscles.

However, if the scale weight is going up, and you start to notice you are more pudgy, and you have to adjust your belt, or your pants are getting tight, then you are probably gaining fat. In that case, you probably want to lower your carbohydrates back down again. Personally, I would not go below 200 grams of carbohydrates a day, if you must cut out more calories I would do it from fat, but I wouldn't go lower than 30 grams of fat a day because your body does need some fat to function optimally. Going too low in calories can be negative on your health overall, so if you want to lose fat and you have already cut your carbohydrates to 200 grams, your fat to 30 grams, and your protein to 80 grams, then that's about 1,400 calories, which is fairly low. If you still are not losing fat, then you could try increasing exercise, and if that does not work, then I would consult a doctor as there may be a medical reason as to why you are unable to lose fat.

Keep in mind that women tend to lose fat slower than men, and women tend to drop weight on the scale suddenly, not gradually. For example, women may, on average, lose 2 pounds a week. However, even though they are doing everything perfectly to lose 2 pounds a week, they may not lose any weight for three weeks, and on the fourth week they suddenly drop 10 pounds. The reason for this is potentially because women tend to store more water than men. And in reality, they did burn 2 pounds of fat a week, but that fat was replaced with water and therefore the scale didn't budge. Eventually that water weight will flush out of their body and it will be reflected as a big drop on the scale. Keep in mind that a gallon of water weighs 8 pounds. And yes, people can dump a gallon of water a day from their bodies. Some people drink a gallon of water a day, although that is not recommended on The First Diet. It is best to drink to thirst, rather than impose a specific amount of water to drink. Drink the amount of water that makes you feel the best.

If you are on a weight loss plan, and taking in low calories, it is important to dedicate one day a week to get at least double the carbohydrates you normally eat. If you are eating 200 grams of carbohydrates a day normally, try to bring that to 400 grams of carbohydrates, maybe 500 grams a day, once a week. This is for three reasons. Reason one is because increasing carbohydrates gives your body a break from the stress of fat loss. The reduction in stress reduces adrenaline and cortisol, and cortisol increases water retention. Increasing carbohydrates reduces stress hormones, which reduces water retention, which helps you lose weight faster. Reason two is that keeping your calories too low for too long can downregulate your thyroid activity and reduce your metabolism. If you want to keep losing weight at a good pace, you'll want to keep your metabolism strong. Increasing your carbohydrate intake once a week will help your thyroid levels go up, and give your metabolism extra strength. Reason three is that it will keep your sanity levels up. Reducing calories for too long can make you feel deprived, stressed, and miserable, adding one high carb day a week can help keep you happy. The trick to these high carb days is to keep your fat intake low, otherwise you may store too much fat and offset your weight loss efforts.

So, at this point let's recap. We know that keeping our carbohydrates at 200 grams or above is best for our metabolisms. And we know that if we are losing weight—and we don't want to—we can increase our carbohydrates until we maintain our weight. If we are not losing weight and we do want to, then we can increase our exercise or decrease our carbohydrates—but try to not go below 200 grams. If you are eating 200 grams of carbohydrates and are still not losing fat, then you can reduce the fat you eat as well. But as we discussed in detail, it is not advisable to cut out protein, carbohydrates, or fat completely.

Chapter 16

DON'T WORRY ABOUT BEING PERFECT

(Real World Examples)

If you've read this far, you may be suffering a bit from information over-load, but don't worry, we'll fix that. I'm glad you've read to this point because now you should have a much better understanding of how your body utilizes nutrients. You understand the differences between how your body uses carbohydrates like starches and sugar. You understand the different types of protein, and why it's important to diversify your protein sources by eating animals nose-to-tail instead of only eating muscle meat. You understand the distinction between saturated fat, monounsaturated fat, and polyunsaturated fat. You also recognize why it's important to get a sufficient quantity of vitamins and minerals and how the foods in The First Diet make that easier to do. Lastly, you know many grams of carbo-hydrates, protein and fat you can start with as a baseline, and how to adjust from there.

But, let's drive things home a little more. Which foods are included in The First Diet and why? Let's go through each category in more detail, broken down by carbohydrate sources, protein sources and fat sources. This will help cement these ideas in your mind. It will also make using The First Diet easier for you. Here are some common First Diet foods you can find at most any grocery store.

Carbohydrate-rich First Diet foods:

Potatoes: All kinds of potatoes, sweet potatoes, white potatoes, small potatoes, big potatoes. If they're edible, they're on the list. Potatoes are nutrient rich foods and they are good sources of copper, magnesium, manganese, potassium, vitamin C, vitamin B6, vitamin B3 and folate. But that's not all. Potatoes have small amounts of many other vitamins like zinc, vitamin K, vitamin B1, and vitamin B2. Basically, potatoes are a nutritional powerhouse and eating them can make getting to your vitamin and mineral goals easier. Potatoes are technically a starch and are not defined as a sugar by The First Diet.

Other root vegetables: Potatoes are not the only root vegetable that grows in the ground. Carrots, parsnips, onions, leeks, and other types of underground vegetables are also packed with nutrients and flavor.

Fruit: Any type of sugary fruit that you can find; the riper the better. Fruits are significantly high in sugar, which helps speed up your metabolism and keeps your body running efficiently. Fruits are also packed with vitamins and minerals, most specifically vitamin C and potassium. Fruit juice can concentrate these vitamins and minerals even more. Although there is debate about whether tomatoes are a fruit or a vegetable, The First Diet puts them in the fruit category.

Sugar: Refined white sugar is a great addition to The First Diet, as it can help speed up your metabolism and make some food taste better. However, refined white sugar does not contain any vitamins or minerals and should only be added to your diet when you know you have already hit your goals for vitamins and minerals for the day. Honey is a better choice, but although honey technically has a wide variety of vitamins and minerals, the absolute amounts are small. Because of this, honey should also only be added if you are sure you are getting enough vitamins and minerals from other sources.

Leafy greens: Kale and spinach are two great additions to round out the nutrients you can get in The First Diet. Kale and spinach are both rich in vitamin K and have significant quantities of magnesium. Other leafy greens can offer variety and diversity in nutrients as well.

Protein-rich First Diet foods:

Beef and lamb: Any cuts of beef or lamb that you enjoy. Steaks, ribs, chuck roasts, pot roasts, ground meat, whatever you like. Beef and lamb are high in vitamin B12, vitamin B6, iron, phosphorus, selenium and zinc. Beef and lamb are some of the best sources of zinc outside of oysters. Beef and lamb also have low levels of polyunsaturated fat, and a good mix of saturated and monounsaturated fats.

Pasture raised pork and chicken: Pasture raised pork and chicken will help ensure these animals do not contain too high levels of polyunsaturated fats. Pasture raised animals also have greater levels of vitamins and minerals, as compared to factory-farmed. Pork is similar to beef and lamb in terms of vitamin and mineral content, although pork has higher levels of vitamin B1 than beef and lamb. Chicken has less iron, less zinc, and more vitamin B3 than beef and lamb.

Gelatin: You can get gelatin in powder form and add it to foods; this is how Jell-O and marshmallows are made. Or you can make a gelatinous broth. Gelatin in powder form does not contain any vitamins and minerals. Instead, it is similar to refined foods in that way. However, gelatin is pure protein and contains the amino acid glycine, which is hard to find outside of gelatin. Making a broth will give you pure gelatin with the addition of vitamins and minerals. The most gelatin-rich broths are made with chicken feet, pig feet, or cow feet.

Liver: You can get liver fresh in the store, then cook it and eat it. Otherwise you can purchase liver pills, but just make sure to get the liver pills that still contain fat. The defatted versions do not have vitamin A. Liver is the best source of vitamin A found anywhere in nature, and also contains high levels of all the B vitamins. In addition, liver is a good source of copper, iron, and vitamin K2. Liver is a nutritional powerhouse.

Pasture raised eggs: Pasture raised eggs are better-tasting and more nutrient dense than factory-farm raised eggs, and next to liver, pasture-raised eggs are the second most concentrated form of vitamins and minerals. In fact, eggs are almost exactly the same as liver in terms of vitamin and mineral composition, but are just less potent. You would need to eat half a dozen eggs to get the same nutritive punch as one ounce of beef liver. However, eggs contain high levels of choline, which is difficult to find outside of eggs in significant levels.

Shellfish: Shellfish like mussels, clams and oysters contain large amounts of vitamins and minerals in a small package. Mussels and clams are full of selenium, vitamin B12, and iron. Oysters are potentially the most concentrated source of zinc in nature, and are also rich in selenium, vitamin B12, and copper.

Fish: Warm water, or whitefish, with low polyunsaturated fat like halibut, cod, rockfish, and tuna are a great way to liven up your protein intake. Fish also contain significant levels of selenium.

Milk (optional): Milk was not available to our tropical African ancestors, but they likely also had access to foods with more calcium and magnesium than we have today. If you can tolerate milk, it can be a great way to easily increase your calcium and magnesium, while getting a protein boost as well. Milk also includes dairy products such as cheese.

Fat-rich First Diet foods:

Coconut oil, olive oil, and butter: These three sources are rich in saturated and monounsaturated fats. Coconut oil is almost completely saturated fat. Butter is mostly saturated fat, and olive oil is almost completely monounsaturated fat. These fat sources are fairly devoid of vitamins and minerals, and because of their lack of vitamins and minerals, they should be used sparingly in The First Diet. But they are absolutely acceptable to incorporate regularly, just not in large quantities.

Chocolate (optional): Any type of chocolate will do, but the more pure the chocolate source the better. Avoiding extra ingredients like soy lecithin, PGPR, and artificial flavors is a good idea. The closer the ingredient list is to "cocoa beans and sugar," the better. Speaking of ingredients, chocolate is mostly saturated fat, with a significant portion of monounsaturated fat, and a tiny bit of polyunsaturated fat. The amount of sugar will depend on the type of chocolate you get, how dark the chocolate is, and the recipe the manufacturer uses.

Animals: Depending on the cut you choose, animals can contain a significant quantity of fat. Ruminant animals like cows and sheep contain mostly saturated and monounsaturated fat, and pasture-raised pigs and chickens contain saturated and monounsaturated fat. However, factory-farm raised chicken and pigs contain significant quantities of polyunsaturated fat and should be minimized.

Bonus First Diet foods:

Coffee: Espresso, drip, French press, latte, mocha, or cappuccino. Pretty much any type of coffee drink includes ingredients found in The First Diet. For example, a mocha is coffee plus milk, sugar, and chocolate. A latte is just coffee and milk. Whatever type of coffee you enjoy the most is best.

Bell peppers: Green, red, orange and yellow, they all grow great in warmer temperatures and are high in vitamin C. They are almost like a low calorie fruit.

Squashes: Pumpkins, butternut squashes, and anything you can find in a grocery store that looks like them. They are similar to root vegetables and are almost like lower calorie potatoes.

Avocados: You can find avocados year round in most grocery stores. Avocados grow well in tropical environments and are mostly made of monounsaturated fat with small amounts of saturated and polyunsaturated fat. Avocados contain a significant amount of B vitamins, copper, vitamin E and vitamin K. Keep in mind that avocados are high in fat, and one avocado can contain close to 30 grams of fat, depending on how big it is.

Mushrooms: Many varieties of wild mushrooms can still be found in Ethiopia and the surrounding areas. Mushrooms, especially wild mushrooms, can hold a significant amount of antioxidants. In addition, mushrooms also contain B vitamins, copper and selenium.

Nuts: There are not many edible nuts and seeds that grow in the tropics. Most of the nuts we see on the shelves today grow in cooler weather away from the equator and therefore contain significant amounts of polyunsaturated fat. If you want to include nuts in your diet, nuts with more stable fats like macadamia nuts, which contain mostly monounsaturated fats, are best for The First Diet. Seeds should be minimized due to the high amounts of polyunsaturated fats.

That leaves us with this list of foods:

- Potatoes (any kind, white potatoes, sweet potatoes, big potatoes, small potatoes, etc.)
- Other root vegetables (onions, carrots, leeks, garlic, etc.)
- Leafy greens
- Fruit (any kind, the riper the better, the sweeter the better)
- Sugar
- Honey
- Coconut oil
- Olive oil
- Butter
- Eggs (pasture raised)
- Shellfish (oysters, mussels, clams, etc.)
- Fish (warm water fish or low fat whitefish like halibut, cod, rockfish, tuna, etc.)
- Animals nose-to-tail (bone broths, gelatin, and liver)
- Milk (and other dairy products like cheese)
- Chocolate
- Coffee
- Bell peppers
- Squashes
- Mushrooms
- Avocados
- Minimal nuts

So now that we have a list of foods, how do we eat them? First let's talk about preparation. It is important to know how to cook each type of food in order to help maximize their nutrient qualities.

Cooking vegetables: (plants)

To begin, let's discuss vegetables. This includes all root vegetables, squashes, and leafy greens. Cooking them well helps maximize your body's ability to absorb their nutrients. This may be common sense to you, but your body would have a hard time digesting a raw potato. That same logic applies to kale, spinach, and any almost any other type of vegetable.

This is because a vegetable's cell walls are made of cellulose, and humans are not designed to break down cellulose well. Cows and sheep can use their four stomachs to digest cellulose, and some other animals can utilize cellulose, too. Humans cannot use cellulose well, and our stomachs cannot destroy the structure of cellulose—that is a big reason why we need to cook our vegetables—to break down the cellulose. Many nutrients are trapped inside the cell walls of plants, and if you do not break down those walls through cooking, then the nutrients will stay trapped inside the plant cell and never be digested by your body. That means those plant nutrients will not be absorbed into your body if they are not broken down. If you want to maximize the amount of vitamins and minerals you are getting, then cooking vegetables is a must.

Cooking muscle meat: (including eggs and shellfish.)

Muscle meat, shellfish and eggs must be cooked until it's safe to eat. Please consult with the USDA guidelines for the exact temperatures each type of meat should be cooked to in order to be safe. Generally speaking, beef and lamb need less cooking than chicken and pork, and eggs should be cooked until the whites are solid. In terms of nutrient absorption, cooking meat to the minimum safety temperatures will maximize absorption. Our human bodies can break down meat much easier than cellulose.

Cooking gelatin:

Gelatin is found in tougher cuts of meat, or in the connective tissues and joints of animals. In order for gelatin to soften enough to eat, connective tissues, joints and tougher cuts of meat need to be cooked for long periods of time at lower heat. Slow cookers work well here, or simmering a bone broth for hours will give you the best results.

Cooking the rest is up to you:

For example, coffee beans usually come precooked, while bell peppers can be eaten raw as a garnish or cooked into an omelette. Mushrooms can be eaten raw or simmered into a stew. Sugar, honey, milk, avocados, nuts and oils usually need no cooking, or have already been pasteurized (heated) before arriving at the store.

Now we have a good list of foods, but how much of each do we eat, and how do we put this together into a cohesive plan?

The first step to make The First Diet work is to know there's no such thing as perfect. If you try to be "perfect," then the chances are high you will become stressed. You'll wonder whether or not you're eating the right foods, maybe you're eating too much or too little of them. The whole point of The First Diet is to help your metabolism and body stay stable, healthy and strong, and stress reduction is a huge part of that. If you start stressing about being perfect, then that defeats the entire purpose of The First Diet. Stressing about a specific food, or meal, could very well make that meal "unhealthy" even if the ingredients themselves are healthy, just because of the stress you're causing your body by worrying.

Therefore, the first step is to relax. You don't need to only eat foods that are in The First Diet. Yes, it's a good idea to lower polyunsaturated fats, but if you go out to eat with friends and you're sure the restaurant uses polyunsaturated-rich soy oil, just eat and be merry. Stressing about soy oil at dinner with your friends is unhealthier than just forgetting about it. In this case, just have fun and eat the soy oil.

Your results from The First Diet will come from what you do on average, and regularly. Your results will come from the rule, not the exception. However, if the exception becomes the rule, then you may be going down the wrong path. Again, it's all about balance, and understanding there is no perfection. Trying to be perfect can destroy you faster than going with the flow when you need to.

Having said that, we know we should try and eat:

Carbohydrates (men and women):

- 200 grams minimum
- 300 grams average
- 300+ depending on activity and muscle mass.

Protein (men and women):

- Minimum of 80 grams.
- Maximum of 1 gram per pound of your bodyweight. (If you're trying to build muscle.)
- Optimum, 100 grams.

Fat:

- Women 55 grams
- Men 65 grams

How exactly do we know if we've gotten 200, 300, or more grams of carbohydrates? How do we know if we've gotten 80, 100, or more grams of protein? And how do we know if we've gone under or over our fat gram goals?

The answer is not fun, but it is true. You need to start tracking your food intake. You must start a food journal, preferably an online food journal that tracks carbohydrates, protein, fat, plus vitamins and minerals. That means you will need to measure, weigh, and enter every piece of food you eat all day long into the food journal you choose. This is not exciting, believe me. I know because I've done it, and I've done it for years.

The good news is that you likely won't need to track your food intake for years if you don't want to. Why? Because, eventually, if you measure, weigh and track every food you eat, every day, eventually you will start to have "x-ray" vision into foods. You will suddenly look at a chicken breast and know just about how much it weighs, how much protein, fat and carbohydrates are in it, without even trying. It becomes kind of like learning to read. Eventually you just look at a word and know what it means without even trying. That's what food journaling will do for you if you stick with it long enough.

Food journaling will show you if you're over or under for specific categories of foods—whether it's carbohydrates, protein or fat. If you see that you've hit your fat goals for the day, and also your protein goals, but you need 30 grams more carbohydrates, it is good to know how to bump that up and reach your goal. The easiest way to do that is to look into the carbohydrate rich category foods we went over earlier in this chapter and choose one of those. For example, you could eat some fruit, drink some fruit juice, or maybe have a leftover small potato.

Things get trickier when you are short on all three types of macronutrients. For example, let's say you were short 15 grams of protein, 10 grams of carbohydrates and 5 grams of fat. It can be difficult to figure out how to fill in those gaps; because, what can you eat, and how much should you eat in order to hit all of those numbers? Finding the right combination of foods that fits in exactly right can be tough at first.

Sometimes you're just kind of stuck, and you won't be able to hit your number perfectly on point. You can either be OK with eating something and going a little over your goal, or deciding you're not hungry and stop eating for that day. But the more you use your food journal, the more you can see opportunities to fill in little gaps like this. For example, to fill in the gap of 15 grams of protein, 10 grams of carbohydrates and 5 grams of fat, you could have a glass of 2% milk. That would get you 5 grams of fat, 12 grams of carbohydrates, and 8 grams of protein. You would then exactly hit your fat goal, and have gone over by 2 grams of carbs, and have 7 grams of protein left. That's not exactly on target, but it's about as close as you'll ever get.

In case you're wondering, I did not engineer that milk example beforehand. I came up with some arbitrary protein, fat, and carbohydrate numbers to target, and then challenged myself to come up with a solution while writing. If you food journal for long enough, you'll start to see opportunities to fill in gaps easily. You'll also be able to accurately estimate how many carbohydrates, protein, and fat you've eaten in a day, without ever having to enter it in a food journal. That skill takes time and practice, but you can do it, and it's worth the process.

The bottom line is that you must keep an online food journal, and you'll need to get familiar with what a day that has 200, 300, or 400 grams of carbohydrates looks and feels like. You'll need to get accustomed to what a day with 80, 100, or 150 grams of protein resembles. And you'll need to be able to recognize what a day with 40, 50, or 70 grams of fat approximates. Then you'll want to cross reference to see if you're getting enough vitamins and minerals. The good news is, due to current technology in online nutritional journals, keeping track is easier than it may seem, especially with some practice. You've just got to give it a try.

Remember to keep stepping on the scale every single morning, and adjust your carbohydrates upwards or downwards to increase or decrease weight. If you want to build muscle, increase both carbohydrates and protein to the appropriate levels. But keep your fat intake at the same basic level. There is no need to increase fat for most people, and increasing fat will likely result in faster fat gain.

But keep in mind that there is no reason to rely 100% on the foods in The First Diet. To keep your metabolism running stable and strong, it is a good idea to gravitate toward the foods in The First Diet, but it is not mandatory that you only use these foods. If you get sufficient amounts of vitamins and minerals in your diet for the day (and The First Diet makes this easy), then you can venture outside of The First Diet for diversity. Examples of this would be white or brown rice, wheat, bread, flour or corn. I would not personally recommend including many polyunsaturated sources, but diversity in carbohydrate sources is completely acceptable if you enjoy it and it agrees with you. However, remember to keep sugar from fruit and other sources as a significant amount of your carbohydrate intake.

So what does an average day look like with The First Diet? Everyone is different, and has unique preferences, so each day will vary from person to person. Finding foods that fit in The First Diet should not be difficult, as The First Diet gives you the option to rely on sugar, starch and saturated fat. Those are common and tasty food sources. It is likely you could think of many recipes you enjoy that would fit The First Diet nicely. But it would still be helpful to see an entire day presented so you can observe a practical application. For example purposes, I'll show you an average day for myself on The First Diet.

An average day for me on The First Diet:

Breakfast:

First Diet Coffee: (full recipe explained in the recipes chapter)

- Honey
- Gelatin
- 2% milk
- Drip coffee

- Oatmeal + brown sugar
- Dried liver pills

Between breakfast and lunch:

- Two cups of drip coffee with sugar
- 1 ½ cups of orange juice

Lunch:

Burrito bowl

- White rice
- Bell peppers
- Onions
- Slow cooked beef
- Salsa
- Sour cream
- Cheese

Between lunch and dinner:

- 1 ½ cups of 2% milk
- Quarter bar of dark chocolate

Dinner:

- Baked potato-fries with a coating of coconut oil
- Chutney and cheese stuffed chicken breast

Before bed:

- 1 cup of orange juice

I should mention that I weigh about 150 pounds, and that amount of food brings me to a grand total of 2,350 calories for the day.

Looking at my food log for these foods, it shows that I have:

- 306 grams of carbohydrates
- 130 grams of protein
- 67 grams of fat

I'm a tiny bit over, by 2 grams on my fat for the day, but that's absolutely fine by me. You won't always hit the bullseye consistently, but getting close is what matters.

And my fat composition for the day was:

- Saturated fat = 35 grams
- Monounsaturated fat = 19 grams
- Polyunsaturated fat = 5 grams

That's about exactly where I want it. Mostly saturated, then comes monounsaturated, and lastly just a little bit of polyunsaturated.

And I diversified my protein intake by choosing a slow-cooked, tougher piece of beef, with more connective tissue and gelatin than a steak. Plus, I added gelatin to my morning coffee. And I took liver pills. That way I am eating nose to tail, including organ meats.

Here's the breakdown for this day's vitamins and minerals:

- Vitamin B1 = 126%
- Vitamin B12 = 881%
- Vitamin B2 = 220%
- Vitamin B3 = 287%
- Vitamin B5 = 186%
- Vitamin B6 = 301%
- Folate = 119%
- Vitamin A = 253%
- Vitamin C = 301%
- Vitamin D = 106%
- Vitamin E = 26%
- Vitamin K = 21%

- Calcium = 112%
- Copper = 482%
- Iron = 212%
- Magnesium = 96%
- Manganese = 142%
- Phosphorus = 273%
- Potassium = 101%
- Selenium = 233%
- Sodium = 77%
- Zinc = 141%

That's a pretty good readout for vitamins and minerals for the day. Vitamin E was low, but we know it's alright to have a little low vitamin E if your polyunsaturated fats are low as well—and mine were low at only 5 grams. My sodium (salt) was also under 100%, but I didn't add in the salt I put on my food in my food journal, so I'm sure that salt is a little higher in reality. I want my salt intake to be at least at 100%, if not more, as salt is an important element of metabolism. Lastly, I was low in vitamin K, but that's OK because later in the week I'll plan on eating more leafy greens, but I didn't have any this day.

Along with remembering to include leafy greens later this week, I'll plan to incorporate some shellfish as well. I'll also add some days with eggs. Not every day needs to include every food in The First Diet. Averages are more important, and as you can see, even without all of the foods, you can still hit over 100% on most of your vitamins and mineral requirements every day.

You may ask why I added orange juice right before bed. I often put some salt in my hand, and wash it down with a glass of orange juice, then rinse with water to protect my teeth. That will boost my salt intake up, and I find it helps me sleep better at night.

One important note about sugar: Fruit, juice or any acidic or sugary substance can promote tooth decay, and it is a smart idea to swish with water after eating or drinking any sugary or acidic foods or drinks. A water rinse in your mouth helps to dilute the sugar and acid on your teeth and can help prevent cavities. Also, remember to brush and floss your teeth regularly. But brushing right after eating or drinking can cause more harm than good as the brush can push sugar and acid into your teeth. It can be better to swish with water and then wait some time before brushing. Our tropical African ancestors did not have toothbrushes, but likely kept their teeth clean by chewing on sticks and roots, which acted very much like brushing and flossing. A high sugar and acid diet means you'll need to be even more careful to keep up proper dental hygiene habits.

One trick I use that helps keep my fat intake on the lower side is to eat mostly fat-free foods in the morning, that way I have more room for fat-rich foods later in the day. For illustration, in the previous example, I started my day with First Diet Coffee and a bowl of sugary oatmeal. Those two have virtually no fat in them and therefore my breakfast is essentially fat free. Then between breakfast and lunch I had coffee with sugar, and orange juice, neither of which have any fat in them. So by lunch I have eaten virtually no fat at all. That frees up many more possibilities for lunch and dinner. Another trick to keeping fat intake down is to get 1% or 2% milk if you're including milk in The First Diet.

And that's really it. If the majority of the foods you eat come from The First Diet, then that will help will help keep your metabolism strong, and your energy levels up. Remember, a healthy metabolism is the foundation to a healthy body.

Before we end this chapter, you should know that there is a possibility that you will feel more tired after eating increased carbohydrates and sugar, especially if you have been avoiding them for some time. This is because when you do not eat enough carbohydrates your stress levels go up in order to compensate, as we discussed earlier in the chapter on stress. Stress hormones can create a feeling of energy, of being excited, or maybe even motivated.

There is an entire industry built around creating artificial stress hormones in the form of drugs that will make you feel more energy, but this energy is at the expense of your health. It is stress energy, not true energy built from a strong and healthy metabolism. Eating enough carbohydrates, especially sugar, can lower those stress hormones, almost instantly, and essentially "pull the rug out" of your stress hormones. When those stress hormones suddenly lower, then you are left at your true energy levels. If your genuine energy level is "tired," then you are likely to feel tired when you eat carbohydrates, especially sugar. And when you avoid carbohydrates, particularly sugar, then your stress hormones will increase, and you will feel that adrenaline energy again.

If you've been avoiding carbohydrates then at some point you may feel dependent on your stress hormones. I know because I've been there, and it's not fun. The dependence is difficult because when you decrease carbohydrates, your stress levels go up and you feel energy, and when you eat carbohydrates, your stress levels crash and you can feel truly tired from all that stress. That is confusing, and can appear that carbohydrates are creating an energy crash. If you believe that, then it seems the only answer is to continue avoiding carbohydrates so you can keep your stress elevated, and your energy high.

This is not a good cycle to be in. We should be lowering our stress hormones, not be dependent on high levels of stress to create energy. But if you find yourself in this cycle, and if you stick with increased carbohydrates, you may be tired at first. But eventually, and likely, you will feel real, authentic, metabolic energy start to increase within you. This undeniable energy will not originate from unhealthy stress hormones; this authentic energy will come from a normal carbohydrate metabolism—and you can get there. Of course, if you are a diabetic, or have serious health complications, this process of restoring normal carbohydrate metabolism, and energy, should be supervised by your doctor. But it will be worth it.

RECIPE EXAMPLES

Now we know what foods are included in The First Diet, and how to find out how much to eat. But very few people want to eat isolated foods exclusively, like dining on an orange with a potato and some ground beef. That's just weird. People want to combine foods into recipes. Recipes create more pleasurable experiences, and we should not eat just for nutrition, we should also eat for pleasure.

So how do we put this together into some recipes? Well, I'm sure you can think of some you already enjoy from the ingredients in The First Diet, but here are some examples for you with approximate nutritional breakdowns as well.

First Diet Coffee

First Diet Coffee is a great addition to the morning. I have been drinking it for years. It is an energy-packed, caffeine-infused protein and sugar drink that relies heavily on gelatin to help round out your protein diversity early in the day. But making it is a tiny bit tricky at first, so here's the breakdown.

Ingredients:

- 20 grams of gelatin (two heaping tablespoons)
- 40 grams of honey or sugar (I prefer honey)
- A splash of milk

Directions:

Put the gelatin powder in a coffee mug, then put honey or sugar in the same mug. Next, mix the sugar or honey together with the gelatin, until combined.

Sugar is easier to combine here, as honey gets kind of gooey. If you're using sugar, just mix until all the granules of sugar and gelatin are combined. If you're using honey, keep mixing until all the dry gelatin is absorbed by the honey. (A metal spoon works well here.)

Next, pour a little coffee over the top of the gelatin and honey/sugar mixture and stir until it starts to melt into the coffee. Pour a little more coffee on top, then mix again, keep pouring coffee and stirring until the entire gelatin honey/sugar mixture is liquefied into the coffee.

Once the mixture is dissolved into the coffee, pour enough milk on top where it cools down the coffee but not so much that it becomes cold. You'll have to experiment with what works the best for you.

This mixture of gelatin, sugar and coffee will help your morning start off right with lots of steady, long-lasting energy without the coffee "crash" that many people experience. The reason there is no crash is because the absorption of the caffeine in the coffee is slowed down by the gelatin to give you balanced energy. In addition, this mixture will enliven you for hours due to the carbohydrate power from the sugar. Finally, the gelatin keeps the carbohydrate energy release nice, slow, and steady.

Nutrition Information per Serving:

- Carbohydrates: 40 grams
- Protein: 20 grams
- Fat: 1 gram

Fish Tacos

Cod fish tacos with fruit salsa (peach, strawberry, jalapeno, cilantro, lime juice), and yogurt ancho chili lime sauce.

Ingredients (two servings)

- 1 ripe peach (diced)
- 8 strawberries (sliced)
- 1/2 a deseeded jalapeno (minced)
- 1 lime
- A small handful of cilantro (chopped)
- Honey-vanilla Greek fat-free yogurt (6 oz.)
- Ancho powder
- 3/4 pound of cod (or white flaky fish)
- 6 corn or flour tortillas

Directions:

Preheat your oven to 350 degrees. Put the cod in a baking pan, and place in the oven for about 15-20 minutes until cooked through and flaky. Meanwhile, mix together the fruit, jalapeno, lime juice, and cilantro. In a separate bowl, mix the yogurt and a teaspoon of ancho powder (or more to taste).

Take out the fish, and flake it apart with a fork, removing all bones. Warm the tortillas up. Take the warm tortillas and put a small layer of the yogurt mixture on the tortillas and spread around. Place the cod on top, and finally add the fruit mixture. Serve.

Nutrition Information per Serving:

- Carbohydrates: 62 grams
- Protein: 43 grams
- Fat: 4 grams

Root Beer Short Ribs and Potatoes

Ingredients (four servings)

- 1 pound short ribs
- 2 carrots (sliced)
- 3 stalks celery (sliced)
- 3 Roma tomatoes (diced)
- 1 medium yellow or sweet onion (diced)
- 78 ounces of tomato paste
- 1 can/bottle root beer
- 4 russet potatoes
- 1 tbsp butter
- 1 tsp coconut oil
- 2 tbsp Sour cream

Directions:

Preheat your oven to 400 degrees. Heat a large skillet with a top (or a Dutch oven) with coconut oil, to medium-high heat. Then salt and pepper the short ribs, and place them into the pan. Sear/brown them evenly, and set aside. Next drain any excess fat, but leave enough to sauté the vegetables in. Put the vegetables into the pan and cook until slightly tender. Add the root beer, the tomatoes, tomato paste, and the short ribs into the skillet or Dutch oven, with the top on, and place in the oven.

Let cook for 2.5 to 3 hours, checking every hour or so, if the liquid gets too low, add a bit of water. Meanwhile, rinse the potatoes, poke some holes in them with a fork or knife and coat with butter, and then roll in salt with a generous layer.

Place the potatoes in a baking pan, and put in the oven when there is about 1.5 hours left of cooking time with the short ribs, so they both come out cooked at the same time. When done, serve the short ribs, and cut open the potatoes and garnish however you would like. Obviously, butter, pepper and sour cream work well.

Nutritional Information per Serving: (will depend on how big the potatoes are and how you garnish them)

- Carbohydrates: 70 grams
- Protein: 30 grams
- Fat: 16 grams

Shellfish Chowder

Ingredients (4 servings)

- 4 large sized Yukon gold potatoes (diced into small squares)
- 1 tbsp butter
- 2.5 pounds of mixed and deshelled seafood (mussels, shrimp, calamari, oysters, white fish, etc.)
- Creamed corn
- 1 bottle of clam juice
- 8 ounces of half and half
- 24 tbsp of flour (to thicken the chowder)
- 16 ounces of chicken broth
- 1 medium sweet or yellow onion (finely diced)

Directions:

Place the bacon on a foil-covered cookie sheet in the oven at 400 degrees until slightly crispy (around 15 minutes). In a large pot or Dutch oven, warm up the butter on medium heat and place in onions. Sauté them until they're translucent.

Add the potatoes, clam juice and chicken broth, and cook on a medium boil until the potatoes are tender. Turn down the heat to medium-low and pour in the seafood and cook until done.

In a separate bowl, combine the flour and half and half, and stir until smooth. Add the mixture to the chowder, and take care to not cook at too high of a heat where the half and half scorches.

Add more flour and half and half if you need it thicker. Add salt and pepper to taste. Serve.

Nutritional Information per Serving:

- Carbohydrates: 57 grams
- Protein: 52 grams
- Fat: 14 grams

CHAPTER 17: RECIPE EXAMPLES

Coconut Oil and Salt Crusted Potato

This is a recipe my wife Lindsey created. It's simply the best way to make a baked potato I've seen. It ends up nice and salty on the outside with a perfectly crispy crust. This recipe is only for the baked potato itself and is not the "dressing" of sour cream, butter or whatever else you'd like to put on it. The dressing is up to you and what you like best.

Ingredients: (2 servings)

- 2 large russet potatoes
- 1 tablespoon coconut oil
- 2 tbsp kosher salt

Directions:

Preheat the oven to 425 degrees. Poke a few holes in each potato with a knife or fork. Place the potatoes in a baking pan, and coat them with the coconut oil until the potatoes are completely covered. Next, sprinkle the salt over the potatoes until they are completely covered. Then put the potatoes in the oven for an hour, or until tender. Remove the potatoes from the oven, and dress them with whatever you'd like.

Note: Lots of the salt and coconut oil will fall to the bottom of the pan while the coconut oil melts in the oven. But just enough salt should be left over to make the skin nicely seasoned.

Nutritional Information per Serving:

- Carbohydrates: 63 grams
- Protein: 6 grams
- Fat: 7 grams

Apple Cider Pork Tenderloin

Ingredients: (4 servings)

- 1 tbsp coconut oil
- 1.5 pounds boneless center cut pork loin, trimmed and tied
- Salt and pepper to taste
- 1 medium onion yellow or sweet (diced)
- 2 carrots (sliced thick)
- 2 stalks celery (sliced thick)
- 3 cloves garlic (smashed)
- 3 sprigs fresh thyme
- 3 sprigs fresh rosemary
- 2 tablespoons cold unsalted butter
- 2 apples (peeled, cored and cut into 8 slices)
- 2 tablespoons apple cider vinegar
- 1 cup apple cider
- 2 tbsp whole grain mustard
- 1 tsp ground coriander
- 1 tsp ground cinnamon
- 1 tsp ground cumin
- 1 tsp cayenne pepper (optional)

Directions:

Preheat the oven to 400 degrees. In a large skillet with a top, or Dutch oven, heat the oil over high heat. Season the pork loin all over generously with salt and pepper. Sear the meat until golden brown on all sides, about 2 to 3 minutes per side.

Transfer the meat to a plate and set it aside. Add the onion, carrot, celery, garlic, herb sprigs, and 2 tablespoons of the butter to the skillet. Stir until the vegetables are browned, about 8 minutes. Stir in the sliced apples, then push the mixture to the sides and set the pork loin in the middle of the skillet along with any collected juices on the plate. Transfer the skillet to the oven and roast the loin until a thermometer inserted into the center of the meat registers 140 to 150 degrees, about 30 to 35 minutes.

Transfer the pork to a cutting board and cover it loosely with foil while you make the sauce. Arrange the apples and vegetables on a serving platter and set aside. Remove and discard the herb sprigs. Return the skillet to a high heat and add the vinegar, scraping the bottom with a wooden spoon to loosen up any browned bits.

Reduce the liquid by half then add the cider and reduce by about half again. Pull the skillet from the heat and whisk in the mustard, and the remaining 2 tablespoons of cold butter. Adjust the seasoning with salt and pepper, to taste.

Remove the strings from the roast and slice into ½ inch thick pieces and arrange over the apple mixture. Drizzle some sauce over the meat and serve the rest on the side.

Nutritional Information per Serving:

- Carbohydrates: 30 grams
- Protein: 38 grams
- Fat: 19 grams

Chicken Broth

This recipe is a great way to get gelatin in your diet, and it tastes great as well. You can use this broth to make rice, or soup, or just drink it straight.

Ingredients: (8 servings)

- 2 pounds of chicken feet
- 2 large carrots, cut in half
- 1 onion, cut coarsely
- 2 celery ribs, cut in half
- 1 bay leaf
- 1 ½ tbsp of salt
- 10 peppercorns

Directions:

Put all of the ingredients into a large pot and pour 2 quarts of water over the ingredients. If it's not enough to cover the ingredients, then pour a little more water in. Bring to a simmer, and cook for at least 3 hours.

Once cooked, strain out all the ingredients and discard them. At this point you should only have broth left. Next, taste a little bit and see if it needs more salt. If it does, then add more salt.

Next, put the broth into a container you can refrigerate and put the container of broth in the refrigerator overnight. The next morning there should be a layer of fat that has congealed at the top. Skim that fat off with a spoon and discard. The broth should feel like Jell-O at this point from all the gelatin in it. Don't worry though. If you reheat it, the gelatin will turn right back into liquid broth while it's warm.

Nutritional Information per Serving:

- Carbohydrates: 0 grams
- Protein: 10 grams
- Fat: 1 gram

Mango Ahi Tuna

Ingredients (2 servings)

- 1 tsp coconut oil
- 1 diced sweet onion
- 1 teaspoon peeled, minced fresh ginger
- 1 teaspoon minced garlic
- 1 ripe mango, peeled, and cut into small pieces
- 4 ounces of canned or fresh pineapple
- 1/3 cup freshly squeezed orange juice
- 2 tsp brown sugar
- 1 tsp salt
- 1/2 tsp freshly ground black pepper
- 1 to 2 tsp minced fresh deseeded jalapeno pepper, or to taste
- 2 tsp minced fresh mint leaves
- 1 tuna steak (3/4 pound)

Directions:

In a large skillet, over medium heat, place the onions with the ginger and garlic and sauté with some coconut oil for about 10 minutes or until the onions are translucent. Turn the stove down to low and put in the mango and pineapple, and cook it all together for about 5-10 minutes.

Next, glug a bit of orange juice in there, with the brown sugar, jalapeno, salt and pepper, then cook for 5-10 minutes (basically until the water from the orange juice mostly evaporates and it gets less soupy).

Finally, add the mint and stir it up. Heat up a pan with some coconut oil at medium heat, but wait awhile, until the oil is moving around in the pan a little like a current. It may even start to smoke a tiny bit.

Sprinkle salt and pepper on either side of the tuna, then place it on the pan. Wait about 30 seconds, then flip it and wait 30 seconds on the other side and take it off the pan. Plate the warm fruit salsa. Cut up the tuna, and put the tuna on top of the warm fruit salsa. Serve.

Nutritional Information per Serving:

Carbohydrates: 47 grams
Protein: 42 grams
Fat: 5 grams

Garlic Mashed Potatoes

Ingredients (4 servings)

- 4 medium russet potatoes (medium size, cubed)
- Enough chicken broth to cover the potatoes (usually around 8-10 ounces)
- 8 cloves of garlic (smashed and diced)
- Salt and pepper to taste
- 2 ounces heavy cream

Directions:

In a medium/large pot, put in the butter and turn to medium-low heat. Take your garlic cloves and smash them hard enough to let some of the inner liquid leak out, and then dice them and place into the heated and buttered pan.

Cook long enough to slightly brown, but don't let them get dark brown. Then place in the cubed potatoes and pour the chicken stock to the point where it's almost covering the potatoes, but some are still sticking out of the liquid. Turn up the heat to a medium boil and cook until the potatoes are fall-apart tender.

A good deal of the liquid should evaporate, but if the liquid is getting far too low and the bottom is burning, add more stock. Once cooked, and most of the liquid is evaporated, take off the heat, and mash with a wooden spatula or potato masher until you get your desired consistency. Leaving some small chunks can add texture.

Next, pour in some heavy cream until the mixture is a bit more hydrated. If it is still not hydrated enough, add some milk. Throw back onto the heat, and stir while it is warming back up to your desired temperature. Salt and pepper to taste. Serve.

Nutrition Information per Serving:

- Carbohydrates: 37 grams
- Protein: 5 grams
- Fat: 8 grams

French Potato Salad

This potato salad is similar to the classic American potato salad, but this version is fresher and not based in mayonnaise. Instead of mayonnaise, it has an olive oil base with white wine vinegar and lots of fresh herbs.

Ingredients:

- 2 pounds of small red potatoes, unpeeled and cut into ¼ inch thick slices
- 2 tsp of salt
- 1 garlic clove that has been peeled and put onto a skewer (metal or bamboo)
- 1 ½ tsp of white wine vinegar
- 2 tsp of Dijon mustard
- ¼ cup of olive oil
- ½ tsp of pepper (black or white)
- 1 small shallot, minced
- 1 ½ tbsp minced fresh parsley
- 1 tbsp minced fresh chives
- 1 ½ tsp minced fresh tarragon

Directions:

Cut 2 pounds of the small red potatoes into ¼ inch thick slices, then put the potatoes and 2 tablespoons of salt in a large saucepan and add enough water to cover them by 1 inch.

Next bring the water with the red potatoes in it to a boil with high heat and reduce the heat to medium. Then put the garlic on the skewer into the hot water, and leave it in there for about a minute to partially cook, then remove it from the water. Immediately run the garlic on the skewer under cold water, and remove the garlic from the skewer and set it aside.

Keep simmering the potatoes until you can stick a knife into and out of the center of a potato slice with no resistance. This should take around 5 minutes. Next, drain the potatoes, but keep ¼ of a cup of cooking water set aside.

Once drained, arrange the hot potatoes close to each other in a single layer on a baking sheet. (You won't be cooking the potatoes more; this just

CHAPTER 17: RECIPE EXAMPLES

so you can evenly season them without tossing them and breaking them apart.)

Press the cooked garlic through a garlic press and put it into a mixing bowl. Alternatively, you could chop up the garlic if you don't have a mincer. Add the minced garlic to the cooked potato water you set aside. Whisk in 1 ½ of a teaspoon of the white wine vinegar, 2 teaspoons of the Dijon mustard, ½ teaspoon of the pepper and ¼ cup of olive oil. Mix it up until it's all combined.

Slowly pour the dressing evenly over the warm potatoes in the baking pan and leave it alone for about 10 minutes. While you are waiting, in another bowl, combine 1 minced shallot, 1 ½ tablespoon of minced parsley, 1 tablespoon of minced chives, and 1 ½ tablespoon of minced tarragon.

Then transfer the potatoes to a large serving bowl and add the shallot and herb mixture. Next, mix it gently together with a rubber spatula to combine. Make sure not to break apart the potatoes when you mix. Serve.

More First Diet Recipes

If you would like more recipes with pictures, please visit:
www.TheFirstDiet.com/recipes

The goal of this book is not to be a recipe collection. The recipes above are more to give you an idea of what recipes you can make with The First Diet. Here are some other easy "go to" foods that fit in as simple snacks or breakfast meals. These don't really need recipes and are fairly self explanatory:

- Cottage cheese and fruit/berries
- Oatmeal
- Chocolate milk
- Greek yogurt and fruit/berries
- Orange juice and eggs
- Fruit, any kind
- Yogurt
- Fruit and cheese
- Etc.

Remember, eating foods like corn, wheat, rice, or other carbohydrate sources is absolutely fine on The First Diet, but it is good to know that these types of foods are best to include if you are certain you will be getting enough vitamins and minerals in your day first. The less nutrient-dense foods should be added in as a bonus, or sprinkled in throughout your day wedged between other nutrient-dense foods or meals. The only food category you should minimize, while on The First Diet, is polyunsaturated fats. I say minimize because you can't completely avoid them, as polyunsaturated fats are found in small amounts virtually everywhere.

Chapter 18

THE FIRST DIET WORKOUTS

The First Diet is mostly focused on nutrition, in an attempt to help you create a healthy, happy, strong metabolism and body. In addition to nutrients, one of the keys to having a healthy, happy, strong metabolism and body is to exercise. No, you don't need to do anything crazy, or intense, but exercise has been shown to have many health advantages. I'm sure you already know that, so I won't waste your time explaining all the potential benefits of exercise, but there are three that I do want to highlight.

Benefit one of working out is that it can help burn fat and keep your weight stable, or help you lose pounds. Even walking can help you burn fat. In fact, lower intensity exercises like walking can specifically target fat burning, whereas higher intensity exercise targets more carbohydrate burning.

Benefit two of working out is that strength training, or training with weights, can help you build muscle, or maintain muscle. Muscle is the biggest influence on how much fat and how many carbohydrates you can burn each day. Fat tissue does not require much energy at all to exist, but muscle needs a great deal of energy to build, and then stick around on your body. If you have more muscle, you can eat more food and not gain fat compared to someone with less muscle.

Benefit three of working out is that it can help boost your mood. Even walking for 30 minutes a day has been shown to help boost people's moods significantly. Strength training can do the same thing. When you have an improved mood, you can make superior decisions, get along better with people, and generally have a greater quality of life.

There is no evidence of our tropical African ancestors' workout routines, but I think it's safe to say that they regularly walked to get food, maybe climbed a tree or two to get fruit, and lifted a few heavy things once in a while. Some of the first human remains in Ethiopia were found alongside the elephants and giraffes they likely hunted and had to bring back to their homes. Elephants and giraffes are very heavy.

So our First Diet workouts are going to be focused on getting around (walking, biking, hiking, climbing) and lifting heavy objects (weights).

The type of workouts you choose should fit in with your lifestyle, your goals, your preferences, and your schedule. Here are some options that translate fairly easy to our modern society.

Walking:

Even walking 30 minutes a day has shown benefits in mood enhancement and will help you burn some fat as well. If you can push this to 60 minutes a day, that's even better if walking is one of your primary workout options.

Weight lifting:

Lifting heavy things can help build your strength and muscle size. Lifting weights can also help you retain muscle while you are losing fat if that's your goal.

If you are below the age of 35 and you recover well, then a strength training routine focused on squats, deadlifts, bench press, military press and other complex big movements can be a good idea if you understand proper form. A good book on this subject is *The Book of Muscle* by Ian King and Lou Schuler.

If you are above the age of 35, or if you do not recover well, then a lighter strength training routine focused on higher reps in the 15-20 rep range can be a better idea for building muscle. Paradoxically, undertraining for people over 35, or for "hardgainers", can be advantageous for muscle gain. For more information on how this works, I recommend reading *The Hardgainer Solution* by Scott Abel.

If you are not familiar with weight training, I suggest you work with a trainer at least until you feel comfortable with the exercises you will be focused on. Find someone who will teach you how to perform the proper technique and form for each exercise. JC Deen is someone I highly trust with both training and nutrition for both males and females.

Bodyweight workouts:

If you don't want to lift weights, but you still want resistance training to build muscle and strength, then bodyweight exercises can work well. I have not personally focused on bodyweight training exclusively, and I do not know the best way to integrate bodyweight exercises into a cohesive plan. However, I have heard good things about a book called *Convict Conditioning* by Paul Wade. It focuses on how convicts are able to build muscle and strength by only using bodyweight techniques. However, I cannot personally vouch for the techniques, as I have not used them.

Sprinting:

It is likely that our tropical African ancestors got themselves into situations they had to get out of quickly. What better way to get out of a situation than to sprint as fast as you can?

Sprinting is an absolute all-out effort, and it can set off some interesting hormonal reactions when you fully exert yourself in that way. Sprinting seems to help people retain their muscle mass better than jogging or running for long periods of time. You only need to look at pictures of marathon runners compared to sprinters and you'll see the difference in muscle mass.

Biking:

Biking is a lot like running or jogging because you'll usually end up biking for fairly long periods of time, and travel many miles when you do. But biking seems to be better than running in terms of metabolic health[1]. This is likely for a few reasons.

Reason one is that your legs are not constantly in motion like when you are running. There are periods of time where you are pedaling your legs, and sometimes when you are coasting downhill, or even coasting on flat road. You don't need to constantly pedal to keep your bike going. Those small rests allow you to have stretches of time where you are able to re-cover for a little bit. Little coasting breaks can make a big difference for your metabolism because you're not beating yourself down for 100% of the time you are moving. You're letting your body "breathe" a bit.

Reason two is that biking is similar to sprinting because sometimes you will need to power up a big hill like a sprint—then you'll get a rest period when you coast back down the hill, just like taking a rest after sprinting. Depending on where you bike, you may be going up and down hills reg-ularly.

Reason three is that biking uses concentric muscle contractions and vir-tually no eccentric muscle contractions. What does that mean? Concentric muscle contractions are when your muscle contracts. Concentric is when you are pushing something away, or standing up, or pulling something toward you.

Eccentric means the opposite of concentric; it's basically opposing a contraction. Eccentric is when you are resisting something that is falling on you, or the motion of sitting down, or preventing a heavy object from falling on the ground. Eccentric is a hard concept to understand, but if you're doing a pushup, the eccentric movement is when you move from up in the air, then down to the ground. The concentric movement is when you push from down on the ground, to up in the air.

Your heart beats exclusively concentrically because it squeezes blood with a concentric pump and then completely relaxes. Your heart does not need to resist any contraction, and therefore it has no eccentric movement. When you only have a concentric movement, you have more endurance, and less muscle soreness, because eccentric movements are what cause most muscle soreness.

Your heart has so much endurance partly because it only beats concen-trically. The same goes for biking. When you bike, you only push the ped-als downward with concentric movements. There's no upwards resistance to create any eccentric action. Another way to think about concentric movements is when you hike up a hill. You are using concentric contrac-tions to go upwards, and when you go back down the hill you are using eccentric movements to keep your legs straight and to keep yourself from falling.

When you use mostly concentric movements, you will get many of the health benefits of exercise, with less muscle soreness, and you can usually last longer without getting exhausted. For example, many people can bike for much longer, and travel further, while still feeling fresh compared to running for the same amount of time or distance. Biking is almost completely concentric movements. Running is a combination of concentric and eccentric.

Rock climbing:

Rock climbing is also mostly a concentric exercise. Climbing is concentric because you're pulling yourself up a rock wall, and then you are lowered down by a rope—not by your own eccentric force.

Aside from being a mostly concentric movement, rock climbing can be fun, and challenging mentally. Many of the routes are as much of a mind puzzle as they are a physical challenge. In fact, at rock climbing gyms, they often call rock climbing routes "problems" because you need to solve them with your brain. You can't always just power through them physically.

Because rock climbing is mostly concentric, you can usually go for longer than you could with other types of exercise that are so reliant on strength. You can also recover faster, which makes it more motivating to go back. In addition, rock climbing can be similar to sprinting in that you will often go all-out with your effort for short periods of time, and then rest for long periods in between climbs. Rock climbing, and climbing in general, would have been a benefit for our tropical African ancestors.

And there we have it, here's the list again of The First Diet workouts:

- Walking
- Weight lifting
- Bodyweight workouts
- Sprinting
- Biking
- Rock climbing

Of course, you should do what works best for you and what you enjoy most. Other great workouts that could apply to The First Diet are martial arts, parkour, fencing, and yoga, but the list goes on. Really, we want to focus on fun activities that fit well in your life, which also build muscle and have built-in rest periods. Long distance running and jogging do not fit well into The First Diet, as they are physically draining, rely heavily on repetitive eccentric movements, and do not have built-in rest periods. If you must run for long periods of time because you enjoy it, that is a valid reason, but make sure to keep your carbohydrates high enough to match your energy needs.

Chapter 19

NUTRITION IS NOT EVERYTHING

Yes, this book discussed the nutritional aspects of The First Diet. This book covered specific foods, carbs, fat, protein, vitamins, minerals and more. But it is important to understand where nutrition fits into the equation of health.

Nutrition can be powerful, but its power is limited. Often diet has more potential to make your health worse than it has the ability to improve your health. The more extreme in any direction you go with diet, the more severe you will be pushing your body, either leaving something out, or adding too much. Either way, you can easily drive your system off balance. One way to go off balance is by focusing your thoughts too much on nutrition and crowding out other important areas of your life.

Because life is a balance, most of what makes you feel happy and enjoy living is not related to the nutrients in your body. Happiness is more related to doing what you enjoy most, feeling important, and spending time with those you love.

And if eating makes you happy, it's not the nutrients in the food that make you feel that way, at least not in the moment. It's the great tasting food that makes you feel happy when you eat. I've never heard someone say, "This hamburger tastes so great because it has 20 grams of fat, 30 grams of protein, and 40 grams of carbohydrates in it!" No, the burger tastes great because the burger tastes great, and someone put a lot of time and thought into making an incredible burger.

Nutrients will never make you happy directly. Sure, nutrients have the ability to enhance your capacity for feeling happy, but mainly by creating a baseline of "not feeling physically bad." For example, if you stop eating, you won't have nutrients coming in, and not eating for an extended period of time will cause you to feel pretty lousy, even a situation that might make you normally feel extremely excited and happy, like going to an amusement park, watching a beautiful sunset, or going to the movies. All of those normally "fun" situations, in the absence of nutrients, will likely be overshadowed by your feelings of hunger. That hunger will likely cause you to be grumpy and upset, or even worried about where your next meal will come from.

In addition, not eating enough, or eating "poorly" for yourself, can lead to some mood disorders like depression. However, it is important to keep in mind that not all physical or mental issues are related to nutrition, and identifying the true cause can be difficult. Trying to fix these types of issues with nutrition alone can be a losing battle.

If you're eating truly destructive foods in enormous quantities—like I did in my fraternity—you may end up with massive headaches, anxiety, or other issues that make doing anything fun impossible for a period of time. Or you could end up with a degenerative disease like Diabetes 2, which could make you feel bad and make enjoying life more difficult.

Generally though, nutrition doesn't have an enormous ability to make you feel any better beyond a baseline of not feeling physically or mentally bad. Once you've hit that baseline, you're done. The rest of your happiness will come from other factors outside of food. But extreme diets have a high likelihood of disturbing your happiness baseline by making you feel physically worse over time, therefore impairing your ability to be happy. If you're not able to be happy, it is likely you will not feel or be healthy, because happiness and healthiness are intimately connected.

There are some who argue that once you've hit your health baseline and you don't feel physically or mentally bad on any significant level, you can still improve because you might be able to extend your lifespan through better diet.

While that may be true, no one has found a predictable way to extend a lifespan, and few people know of any reliable way to even prevent diseases like cancer through diet. Many extreme diets trying to prevent diseases may end up causing other unintended issues. When you treat food like a drug, even food can have side effects.

So, what's the best approach? No one can really answer that question because, like it or not, everyone is different. Each person weighs differently, they have a little more muscle, a little less fat, they may move around more during the day, or exercise at a greater frequency. They may have a stressful work life, or maybe they relax in the sun all day. Some may live at higher altitudes with a little less oxygen in the air. Someone could have genetic variations, allergies, or be exposed to environmental toxins. Basically, no two people are the same, and no two people will respond the same way to one diet.

Although the average size of all rocks on Earth may be 5 centimeters across, there are few actual rocks that are exactly 5 centimeters across. Even the ones close to 5 centimeters will not be precisely 5 centimeters; they will be something like 4.8, 5.1, or 4.98 centimeters. Close, but not exactly 5 centimeters— not exactly average. Average is a concept, not a reality. In reality there are few "exactly average" people, even though statistically there are many average people. Trying to fit into the average mold won't work unless you're one of the weirdly exactly average people. And even if you do fit the exact "average" today, what about in 5 years? Each person is constantly changing, and evolving over time.

It may sound like a boring answer, but moderation and variety make for a smart approach to life and diets. And sometimes you even need moderation in moderation. But when it comes down to it, you have to figure out what works best for you because no one is you, and therefore no one knows what you should do, except you. So the best advice may be to not take anyone's advice at all.

That last statement is pretty much the definition of a paradox. How can you take the advice of not listening to advice? There's no way to do both at the same time, but a wise man once said that paradoxes are the truth standing on its head in order to get attention. Many of life's great truths are hidden in paradoxes, and examining them and getting personal insight from them can be a rewarding exercise. Having said all of this, advice is different from knowledge. Advice is born from knowledge and wisdom. And if you want to give yourself advice—which is probably the best advice possible for you—then you will need knowledge from which to build your own advice.

It is almost impossible to come up with advice for yourself if you don't know any of the basics about nutrition. Asking someone to just "figure it out" can work, but that's asking a lot, and the person who "just figures it out" will have to go through an extended period of trial and error, which can be frustrating and dangerous.

You may have already discovered the optimal way of eating for yourself, but if you think there may be something better out there, you may abandon it while looking for "greener pastures" and only get lost in the process. Someone may even convince you to leave your "nutritional path" and try theirs due to their own personal success. But what worked for them may not work for you. It's just as important to stop while you're ahead as it is to find out how to get ahead in the first place.

This book was written to help you shortcut a big part of your learning curve, and help you formulate your own advice, for yourself. Yes, this book gave some recommendations, but you will ultimately need to create your own path with the knowledge you gained in this book.

Chapter 20

ONE LAST WORD ON THE LIMITATIONS OF DIET

A successful diet is as much psychological as it is physical. This is a huge part of the reason why most diets fail to produce long term results. And that is why you must understand the mind as well as the body. They are connected.

Let's start with a few quick questions. Why are so many people unhealthy? Why can't even those who know how to get healthy seem to take the right actions? Why can't they find the motivation? And why are some people doing everything right, but they can't get their health to turn around?

Of course there are many answers to these questions, but here's a compelling angle. Would you like to know the easiest way to lose muscle mass, bone density, and be virtually guaranteed to huff and puff up a flight of stairs? No, it's not smoking. It's doing nothing. Use it or lose it, atrophy[1].

Yes, that's old news. It's not exciting. You already knew that. But there's something more profound in the truth about atrophy. There's something about the human soul hidden in the atrophy phenomenon. Before we get into that, first you need to know about Howard Bloom.

If you're not familiar with Howard Bloom, you should be. He's not a health writer or researcher specifically, but what he has to say is interesting—and some of it applies directly to your health. You should listen to him because Howard has had, and overcome, a fair share of health issues. Howard had a flourishing career as a publicist for Michael Jackson, ZZ Top, Kiss, AC/DC and a bunch of other famous musicians.

Then one day he couldn't get out of bed. That inability to get out of bed lasted for 15 years. He eventually figured out how to beat his Chronic Fatigue Syndrome, and he's been an active writer, philosopher and activist since.

In Howard's book, The Lucifer Principle, he discusses the subject of atrophy and how it relates to human health in a profound way that you may never expect. I know I didn't. Here it is in a nutshell.

Your body is made of cells. If you don't need those cells, they atrophy away. For example, if a bodybuilder gets huge, and puts on 70 pounds of extra muscle, then stops training, that muscle will disappear quickly. If someone goes into space, their muscles, and bone density starts to fade away—because it's not needed in a zero gravity atmosphere.

Your cells need constant positive feedback. They need to know they are important, or they push the self-destruct button and die. The scientific term for when cells self-destruct is called "apoptosis."

That's right, if a cell feels unimportant, not needed, or ignored, it will literally commit suicide. Why is this important? The human race is like one big organism, and each cell in our organism is a human. You are a cell in the human organism.

Each "human cell" needs positive feedback to feel needed. Each "human cell" must feel important, they must not be ignored. They must not be put down, or made to feel outcast. This is poison to the individual human, just like it is to the cells that make up your body.

That is happening to countless humans across the globe right now. People feel like they are not needed, not important, like if they died right now no one would care. If you feel that way, you better watch out because if you have those feelings, you may be sending out unconscious self-destruct signals to yourself right now.

These self-destruct signals don't include instant suicide for most. But many start to slowly kill themselves from the inside out. It may be eating too much, sitting around too often, watching TV more than you should. Maybe these self-destruct signals come in the form of insane anxiety, or the type of loneliness that won't let you try to become un-lonely. Maybe you self-sabotage, or maybe somehow your body makes you tired, unmotivated, bored, resigned, or apathetic. Maybe that's how your body's self-destruct signals work. If you don't feel important, needed, wanted, or vital, the human default mode is to self-destruct.

So maybe the best thing anyone can do for their health is to find things that make them feel important and needed. Maybe that's your family, or maybe that's your friends. Maybe you want to help teach people to be the best they can be at math, or you could volunteer to be a big brother or sister at a youth center. Maybe that thing isn't even people. Maybe you hate people, and you've been tortured by people your entire life. Well, go find a cause then. Rescue puppies or help restore the environment.

If you feel unimportant, the last thing you should do is sit there and wait. You need to do something right now to change that. The good news is that someone or something is just waiting for you to become important in their lives right now. You can help; you can make a difference, no matter how small, because even the small stuff matters.

Because, if you do that small stuff, and it matters to someone, then you matter. And you should work at mattering because mattering is one of the most important things you can do for your health. No nutrition plan will save you unless you find a way to matter to someone, and let them know they matter to you too.

CONCLUSION

Now more than ever we must take our health back. There is something unusual occurring in our current mainstream health advice. We are being told to completely remove one of the healthiest foods humans can eat: sugar. And then we are asked to include one of the unhealthiest foods for humans: polyunsaturated fat.

Over the past 30 years, what has this advice achieved? It's certainly not helped our obesity epidemic, and in fact it may have started it. The amount of polyunsaturated fat in our tissues has gone up almost exactly inline with the obesity epidemic.

Scientists can see what people have been eating by examining their cells. Studies show that in the year 1960, eight percent of people's fat tissues in the U.S. were made of "cold weather" polyunsaturated fat. In 2008, that number jumped to twenty-five percent.

Now contrast that with the fact that in the year 1960, thirteen percent of people in the U.S. were obese. In 2010, that number increased to thirty-five percent obese. That's a 310% increase in "cold weather" fat in our tissues, and a 270% increase in obesity—a close tie in numbers.

In addition, the total amount of caloric sweeteners eaten in the U.S. took a sharp decline around 1998, and that did nothing to stop the obesity epidemic. From 1998 to 2010, sugar consumption dropped by 15%, and while people in the U.S. were eating less sugar, the number of obese individuals went up by approximately 37%.

We have also seen that our brains evolved in tropical, and tropical-savanna Africa where there were abundant sugar sources. Once the drought forced humans north and south of the tropics, and we had less access to sugar, our brains shrank. We lost a tennis ball-sized chunk of brain mass. Only once the sugar trade came into existence did our brains start growing again.

Something has to change, and The First Diet could be the solution. The First Diet proposes that we continue to eat sugar as a significant source of our caloric intake, preferably from nutrient-dense sources. The First Diet invites us to decrease our polyunsaturated fat intake to help reduce the levels we store in our bodies. The First Diet suggests that we should rely on stable fats, such as saturated and monounsaturated, so we can help support our bodies and metabolisms, all while optimizing our vitamin and mineral intake.

This sounds complex, but the reality is that it is not. We evolved in an environment that gave us the nutrition we needed to evolve. Our ancient tropical environment provided us all of the nutrients we needed to not only survive, but thrive. We thrived so well that we evolved big luxurious brains that take up 2% of our body mass and use 20% of our metabolism. Humans are designed to be high energy beings; we do not do well when we shortchange our metabolisms and rob our bodies of the sugar we evolved with. When warm-blooded humans eat fats designed for cold weather, our bodies begin to go rancid from the inside out.

If we simply rely on the foods that were present 200,000 years ago in the tropics, we can get everything we need from a nutritional standpoint. All of the nutrients that helped our metabolisms evolve to high energy beings are right there in the tropics for our taking. And the good news is now, thanks to our modern society, those tropical foods are available to you in your local grocery store.

Because of this, you can start The First Diet today. Don't put off creating and experiencing the improvement of health you truly want, and deserve, for another day.

MAY I ASK YOU A QUICK FAVOR?

If this book has added value to your life, if you feel like you are better off after reading it, and you see that The First Diet can be a new beginning for you to improve your health, I'm hoping you will do something for someone you care about.

Give this book to them, or let them borrow your copy. Ask them to read it, or better yet, get them their own copy, maybe as a birthday or holiday gift.

If you believe that part of being a great friend or family member is about helping your friends and loved ones to become healthier and happier, I encourage you to share this book with them.

Please spread the word.

Thank you so much.

RDA REFERENCES

RDA for Vitamin A:

Children

- 1 to 3, 1,000 IUs
- 4 to 8, 1,320 IUs
- 9 to 13, 2,000 IUs

Men

- 14 to 18, 3,000 IUs
- 19+, 3,000 IUs

Women

- 14 to 18, 2,310 IUs
- 19+, 2,310 IUs

Pregnant women

- 14 to 18, 2,500 IUs
- 19+, 2,565 IUs

Breastfeeding women

- 14 to 18, 4,000 IUs
- 19+, 4,300 IUs

RDA for B Vitamins:

RDA for B1 (Thiamine):

Infants

- 0 to 6 months, 0.2 mg
- 7 to 12 months, 0.3 mg

Children

- 1 to 3 years, 0.5 mg
- 4 to 8 years, 0.6 mg

Boys

- 9 to 13 years, 0.9 mg

Men

- 14 years and older, 1.2 mg

Girls

- 9 to 13 years, 0.9 mg

Women

- 14 to 18 years, 1 mg
- over 18 years, 1.1 mg

Pregnant women

- 1.4 mg

Breastfeeding women

- 1.5 mg

RDA FOR B2 (RIBOFLAVIN):

Infants

- 0 to 6 months, 0.3 mg
- 7 to 12 months, 0.4 mg

Children

- 1 to 3 years, 0.5 mg
- 4 to 8 years, 0.6 mg
- 9 to 13 years, 0.9 mg

Men

- 14 years or older, 1.3 mg

Women

- 14 to 18 years, 1 mg
- over 18 years, 1.1 mg

Pregnant women

- 1.4 mg

Breastfeeding women

- 1.6 mg

RDA FOR B3 (NIACIN, OR NIACINAMIDE):

Infants

- 0 to 6 months, 2 mg
- 7 to 12 months, 4 mg

Children

- 1 to 3 years, 6 mg
- 4 to 8 years, 8 mg
- 9 to 13 years, 12 mg

Men

- 14 years and older, 16 mg

Women

- 14 years and older, 14 mg

Pregnant women

- 18 mg

Breastfeeding women

- 17 mg

RDA FOR B5 (PANTOTHENIC ACID):

Infants

- 0 to 6 months, 1.7 mg
- 7 to 12 months, 1.8 mg

Children

- 1 to 3 years, 2 mg
- 4 to 8 years, 3 mg
- 9 to 13 years, 4 mg

Men and women

- 14 years and older, 5 mg

Pregnant women

- 6 mg

Breastfeeding women

- 7 mg

RDA FOR B6:

Infants

- 0 to 6 months, 0.1★ mg
- 7 to 12 months, 0.3★ mg

★Adequate intake (AI)

Children

- 1 to 3 years, 0.5 mg
- 4 to 8 years, 0.6 mg
- 9 to 13 years, 1.0 mg

Men

- 14 to 50 years, 1.3 mg
- over 50 years, 1.7 mg

Women

- 14 to 18 years, 1.2 mg
- 19 to 50 years, 1.3 mg
- Over 50 years, 1.5 mg

RDA FOR B7 (BIOTIN):

Infants

- 0 to 12 months, 7 mcg

Children

- 1 to 3 years, 8 mcg
- 4 to 8 years, 12 mcg
- 9 to 13 years, 20 mcg

Adolescents

- 14 to 18 years, 25 mcg

Adults

- Over 18 years, 30 mcg

Pregnant women

- 30 mcg

Breastfeeding women

- 35 mcg

RDA FOR B9 (FOLIC ACID):

Infants

- 0 to 6 months, 65 mcg
- 7 to 12 months, 80 mcg

Children

- 1 to 3 years, 150 mcg
- 4 to 8 years, 200 mcg
- 9 to 13 years, 300 mcg

Men

- 14 and older, 400 mcg

Women

- 14 to 50, 400 mcg plus 400 mcg from supplements or fortified foods
- 50 and over, 400 mcg

Pregnant women

- 600 mcg

Breastfeeding women

- 500 mcg

RDA FOR B12:

Infants

- 0 to 6 months, 0.4 mcg
- 7 to 12 months, 0.5 mcg

Children

- 1 to 3 years, 0.9 mcg
- 4 to 8 years, 1.2 mcg
- 9 to 13 years, 1.8 mcg

Adolescents and Adults

- 2.4 mcg

Pregnant women

- 2.6 mcg

Breastfeeding women

- 2.8 mcg

RDA for Vitamin C:

Infants

- 0 to 6 months, 40* mg
- 7 to 12 months, 50* mg

Adequate Intake (AI)

Children

- 1 to 3 years, 15 mg
- 4 to 8 years, 25 mg
- 9 to 13 years, 45 mg

Girls

- 14 to 18 years, 65 mg

Boys

- 14 to 18 years, 75 mg

Men

- 19 and older, 90 mg

Women

- 19 years and older, 75 mg

RDA for Vitamin D:

Infants

- 0 to 6 months, 400 IUs
- 7 to 12 months, 400 IUs

Children

- 1 to 3 years, 600 IUs
- 4 to 8 years, 600 IUs

Older children and adults

- 9 to 70 years, 600 IUs
- Over 70 years, 800 IUs

Pregnant and breastfeeding

- 600 IUs

RDA for Vitamin E:

Infants

- 0 to 6 months, 4 mg
- 7 to 12 months, 5 mg

Children

- 1 to 3 years, 6 mg
- 4 to 8 years, 7 mg
- 9 to 13 years, 11 mg

Adolescents and Adults

- 14 and older, 15 mg

RDA for vitamin K:

(the RDA does not distinguish between K1 and K2)

Infants

- 0 to 6 months, 2.0 micrograms per day (mcg)
- 7 to 12 months, 2.5 mcg

Children

- 1 to 3 years, 30 mcg
- 4 to 8 years, 55 mcg
- 9 to 13 years, 60 mcg

Adolescents

- 14 to 18, 75 mcg

Adults

- 19 and older, 90 mcg

RDA for Calcium:

Infants

- 0 to 6 months, 200 mg
- 7 to 12 months, 260 mg

Children and Adolescents

- 1 to 3 years, 700 mg
- 4 to 8 years, 1,000 mg
- 9 to 18 years, 1,300 mg

Men

- 19 to 50 years, 1,000 mg
- 50 to 70 years, 1,000 mg
- Over 71 years, 1,200 mg

Women

- 1,200 mg

Pregnancy and Breastfeeding

- 14 to 18 years, 1,300 mg
- 19 to 50 years, 1,000 mg

RDA for Iron:

Infants

- 0 to 6 months, 0.27 mg
- 7 to 12 months, 11 mg

Children

- 1 to 3 years, 7 mg
- 4 to 8 years, 10 mg

Males

- 9 to 13 years, 8 mg
- 14 to 18 years, 11 mg
- 19 to 30 years, 8 mg
- 31 to 50 years, 8 mg
- 51 to 70 years, 8 mg
- 70+ years, 8 mg

Females

- 9 to 13 years, 8 mg
- 14 to 18 years, 15 mg
- 19 to 30 years, 18 mg
- 31 to 50 years, 18 mg
- 51 to 70 years, 8 mg
- 70+ years, 8 mg

Pregnant Women

- 27 mg

Lactating Women

- 14 to 18 years, 10 mg
- 19+ years, 9 mg

RDA for Phosphorus (phosphate)

Infants

- 0 to 6 months, 100 mg
- 7 to 12 months, 275 mg

Children

- 1 to 3 years, 460 mg
- 4 to 8 years, 500 mg
- 9 to 18 years, 1,250 mg

Adults

- 19 years and older, 700 mg

Pregnant and breastfeeding

- Under 18 years, 1,250 mg
- 19 years and older, 700 mg

RDA for Magnesium:

Infants

- – 0 to 6 months, 30 milligrams per day (mg)
- – 7 to 12 months, 75 mg

Children and Adolescents

- – 1 to 3 years, 80 mg
- – 4 to 8 years, 130 mg
- – 9 to 13 years, 240 mg

Males

- – 14 to 18 years, 410 mg
- – 19 to 30 years, 400 mg
- – Over 31 years, 420 mg

Females

- – 14 to 18 years, 360 mg
- – 19 to 30 years, 310 mg
- – Over 31 years, 320 mg

Pregnant women

- – 14 to 18 years, 400 mg
- – 19 to 30 years, 350 mg
- – 31 to 50 years, 360 mg

Breastfeeding women

- – 14 to 18 years, 360 mg
- – 19 to 30 years, 310 mg
- – 31 to 50 years, 320 mg

RDA for Manganese:

No recommended dietary allowances (RDA) for manganese have been established. When there are no RDAs for a nutrient, the Adequate Intake (AI) is used as a guide.

The AI is the estimated amount of the nutrient used by a group of healthy people and assumed to be adequate.

The daily Adequate Intake (AI) levels for manganese are:

Infants

- 0 to 6 months, 3 mcg
- 7 to 12 months, .6 mg

Children

- 1 to 3 years, 1.2 mg
- 4 to 8 years, 1.5 mg

Boys

- 9 to 13 years, 1.9 mg
- 14 to 18 years, 2.2 mg

Girls

- 9 to 18 years, 1.6 mg

Men

- 19 and older, 2.3 mg

Women

- 19 and older, 1.8 mg

Pregnant women

- 14 to 50 years, 2 mg

Breastfeeding women

- 2.6 mg

Tolerable Upper Intake Levels (UL) for manganese, the highest level of intake at which unwanted side effects are not expected, have been established.

The daily ULs for manganese are:

Children

- 1 to 3 years, 2 mg
- 4 to 8 years, 3 mg
- 9 to 13 years, 6 mg
- 14 to 18 years (including pregnant and breastfeeding women), 9 mg

Adults

- 19 years and older (including pregnant and breastfeeding women), 11 mg

RDA for Zinc:

Infants

- 0 to 6 months, 2 mg
- 7 to 12 months, 3 mg

Children

- 1 to 3 years, 3 mg
- 4 to 8 years, 5 mg
- 9 to 13 years, 8 mg

Adolescents

- 14 to 18 years (boys), 11 mg
- 14 to 18 years (girls), 9 mg

Men

- 11 mg

Women

- 8 mg

Pregnant women

- 14 to 18 years, 12 mg
- Over 18 years, 11 mg

Breastfeeding women

- 14 to 18 years, 13 mg
- Over 18 years, 12 mg

RDA for Copper:

Adults

- 0.9 mg

RDA for Selenium:

Infants

- 0 to 6 months, 15 mcg
- 7 to 12 months, 20 mcg

Children

- 1 to 3 years, 20 mcg
- 4 to 8 years, 30 mcg
- 9 to 13 years, 40 mcg

Adolescents and Adults

- 14+ years, 55 mcg

Pregnant women

- 60 mcg

Breastfeeding women

- 70 mcg

RDA for Potassium:

Infants

- 0 to 6 months, 400 mg
- 7 to 12 months, 700 mg

Children

- 1 to 3 years, 3,000 mg
- 4 to 8 years, 3,800 mg
- 9 to 13 years, 4,500 mg

Adult

- 19+ years, 4,700 mg

Pregnant women

- 4,700 mg

Breastfeeding women

- 5,100 mg

RDA for Iodine:

Infants

- 0 to 6 months, not possible to establish
- 7 to 12 months, not possible to establish

Children

- 1 to 3 years, 200 mcg
- 4 to 8 years, 300 mcg
- 9 to 13 years, 600 mcg

Adult

- 14 to 18, 900 mcg
- 19+ years, 1,100 mcg

Pregnant women

- 14 to 18, 900 mcg
- 19+ years, 1,100 mcg

Breastfeeding women

- 14 to 18, 900 mcg
- 19+ years, 1,100 mcg

CHAPTER REFERENCES

Chapter 1: Important: Read this before You Begin

1. Menke A, Rust KF, Fradkin J, Cheng YJ, Cowie CC. Associations between trends in race/ethnicity, aging, and body mass index with diabetes prevalence in the United States: a series of cross-sectional studies. Ann Intern Med. 2014;161(5):328-35.

2. Centers for Disease Control and Prevention. Overweight and Obesity: Adult Obesity Facts.

3. National Institute on Aging, National Institutes of Health, U.S. Department of Health and Human Services, World Health Organization. Global Health and Aging: Pgs. 9-12.

Chapter 2: What this Book Will Show You

1. Stratigraphic placement and age of modern humans from Kibish, Ethiopia. Nature. 2005;433(7027):733.

2. Bradshaw JL. Human Evolution, A Neuropsychological Perspective. Psychology Press; 1997. Pg 185.

3. Scholz CA, Johnson TC, Cohen AS, et al. East African megadroughts between 135 and 75 thousand years ago and bearing on early-modern human origins. Proc Natl Acad Sci USA. 2007;104(42):16416-21.

4. Cane MA, Molnar P. Closing of the Indonesian seaway as a precursor to east African aridification around 3-4 million years ago. Nature. 2001;411(6834):157-62.

5. Mackowiak PA. Temperature regulation and the pathogenesis of fever. In: Mandell GL, Bennett JE, Dolin R, eds. Principles and Practice of Infectious Diseases. 7th ed. Philadelphia, PA: Elsevier Churchill-Livingstone; 2009:chap 50.

6. Bianconi E, Piovesan A, Facchin F, et al. An estimation of the number of cells in the human body. Ann Hum Biol. 2013;40(6):463-71.

7. Witting LA, Lee L. Recommended dietary allowance for vitamin E: relation to dietary, erythrocyte and adipose tissue linoleate. Am J Clin Nutr. 1975;28(6):577-83.

8. Ren J, Dimitrov I, Sherry AD, Malloy CR. Composition of adipose tissue and marrow fat in humans by 1H NMR at 7 Tesla. J Lipid Res. 2008;49(9):2055-62.

9. Centers for Disease Control and Prevention. Overweight and Obesity: Adult Obesity Facts.

10. U.S.D.A. Tables on Sweetener Consumption (Excel).

11. White JS. Challenging the fructose hypothesis: new perspectives on fructose consumption and metabolism. Adv Nutr. 2013;4(2):246-56.

Chapter 4: How the Caveman Diet Took a Chunk out of My Brain the Size of a Tennis Ball

1. Stratigraphic placement and age of modern humans from Kibish, Ethiopia. Nature. 2005;433(7027):733.

2. Affairs OO, Development BO, Council NR et al. Lost Crops of Africa:, Volume I: Grains. National Academies Press; 1996.

3. Cooperation DS, Affairs PA, Council NR. Lost Crops of Africa:, Volume II: Vegetables. National Academies Press; 2006.

4. Cooperation DS, Affairs PA, Council NR. Lost Crops of Africa:, Volume III: Fruits. National Academies Press; 2008.

5. Scholz CA, Johnson TC, Cohen AS, et al. East African megadroughts between 135 and 75 thousand years ago and bearing on early-modern human origins. Proc Natl Acad Sci USA. 2007;104(42):16416-21.

6. Anton Vaks, Miryam Bar-Matthews, Avner Ayalon, Alan Matthews, Ludwik Halicz, and Amos Frumkin. Desert speleothems reveal climatic window for African exodus of early modern humans. Geology, September, 2007, v. 35, p. 831-834

7. Magill CR, Ashley GM, Freeman KH. Water, plants, and early human habitats in eastern Africa. Proc Natl Acad Sci USA. 2013;110(4):1175-80.

8. Pagani L, Kivisild T, Tarekegn A, et al. Ethiopian genetic diversity reveals linguistic stratification and complex influences on the Ethiopian gene pool. Am J Hum Genet. 2012;91(1):83-96.

9. Gonder MK, Mortensen HM, Reed FA, De sousa A, Tishkoff SA. Whole-mtDNA genome sequence analysis of ancient African lineages. Mol Biol Evol. 2007;24(3):757-68.

10. Roebroeks W, Villa P. On the earliest evidence for habitual use of fire in Europe. Proc Natl Acad Sci USA. 2011;108(13):5209-14.

11. Hunter-gatherers and human evolution. Evolutionary Anthropology: Issues, News, and Reviews. 14(2):54.

12. Oppenheimer S. Out-of-Africa, the peopling of continents and islands: tracing uniparental gene trees across the map. Philos Trans R Soc Lond, B, Biol Sci. 2012;367(1590):770-84.

13. Bocquet-appel JP. When the world's population took off: the springboard of the Neolithic Demographic Transition. Science. 2011;333(6042):560-1.

14. Savolainen P, Zhang YP, Luo J, Lundeberg J, Leitner T. Genetic evidence for an East Asian origin of domestic dogs. Science. 2002;298(5598):1610-3.

15. Harlan JR: Crops and Man. Madison, American Society of Agronomy, 1992.

16. Kathleen McAuliffe. "If Modern Humans Are So Smart, Why Are Our Brains Shrinking?" Discover September 2010.

17. Raichle ME, Gusnard DA. Appraising the brain's energy budget. Proc Natl Acad Sci USA. 2002;99(16):10237-9.

18. Cryer PE. Hypoglycemia, functional brain failure, and brain death. J Clin Invest. 2007;117(4):868-70.

19. Lecoultre V, Benoit R, Carrel G, et al. Fructose and glucose co-ingestion during prolonged exercise increases lactate and glucose fluxes and oxidation compared with an equimolar intake of glucose. Am J Clin Nutr. 2010;92(5):1071-9.

20. Kenneth L. Beals, Courtland L. Smith, Stephen M. Dodd. Brain Size, Cranial Morphology, Climate, and Time Machines. Current Anthropology V01. 25, NO 3, June 1984

21. Guyenet, Stephan. "Glucose Tolerance in Non-industrial Cultures". Whole Health Source. November 20 2010. Web. 12 March 2015.

22. Little, Charles E., 1987: Beyond the mongongo tree: good news about conservation tillage and the environmental tradeoff. Journal of Soil and Water Conservation 42: 31

23. Liebenberg L. The relevance of persistence hunting to human evolution. J Hum Evol. 2008;55(6):1156-9.

24. Taylor AB, Van schaik CP. Variation in brain size and ecology in Pongo. J Hum Evol. 2007;52(1):59-71.

25. Northern Territory Government Australia. Department of Health and Community Services. The Bush Book. Volume 2. Chapter 3. "The diet of Aboriginal people before European contact."

26. Terese B. Hart, John A. Hart. The ecological basis of hunter-gatherer subsistence in African Rain Forests: The Mbuti of Eastern Zaire. Human Ecology. 1986;14 (1): 29.

27. Migliano AB, Vinicius L, Lahr MM. Life history trade-offs explain the evolution of human pygmies. Proc Natl Acad Sci USA. 2007;104(51):20216-9.

28. Sheridan RB. Sugar and slavery. Baltimore, MD: The Johns Hopkins University Press, 1973.

29. Stratigraphic placement and age of modern humans from Kibish, Ethiopia. Nature. 2005;433(7027):733.

30. Cooperation DS, Affairs PA, Council NR. Lost Crops of Africa:, Volume III: Fruits. National Academies Press; 2008.

31. Bryan RN, Bilello M, Davatzikos C, et al. Effect of diabetes on brain structure: the action to control cardiovascular risk in diabetes MR imaging baseline data. Radiology. 2014;272(1):210-6.

32. Deaner, R.O., et al. 2007. Overall brain size, and not encephalization quotient, best predicts cognitive ability across non-human primates. Brain, Behavior, and Evolution, 70: 115-124.

33. Aiello, L.C. & Wheeler, P. 1995. The expensive-tissue hypothesis: the brain and the digestive system in human and primate evolution. Current Anthropology, 36: 199-121

34. Marino, L. 1998. A comparison of encephalization between odontocete cetaceans and anthropoid primates. Brain, Behavior, and Evolution, 51: 230-238.

Chapter 5: Why Sugar Is Good for You

1. Taubes, Gary. "Is Sugar Toxic?" The New York Times Magazine. April 17 2011. Page MM47.

2. Sisson, Mark. "Dear Mark: Sugar as Immune Suppressant". Mark's Daily Apple. March 29 2010. Web. 16 March 2015.

3. Melnick, Meredith. "Sugar In Diet Linked To Type 2 Diabetes Rates, Study Finds". Huffington Post. February 28 2013. Web. 16 March 2015.

4. Boggiano MM, Dorsey JR, Thomas JM, Murdaugh DL. The Pavlovian power of palatable food: lessons for weight-loss adherence from a new rodent model of cue-induced overeating. Int J Obes (Lond). 2009;33(6):693-701.

5. Garber AK, Lustig RH. Is fast food addictive?. Curr Drug Abuse Rev. 2011;4(3):146-62.

6. Acheson KJ, Schutz Y, Bessard T, Anantharaman K, Flatt JP, Jéquier E. Glycogen storage capacity and de novo lipogenesis during massive carbohydrate overfeeding in man. Am J Clin Nutr. 1988;48(2):240-7.

7. Nelson DL, Lehninger AL, Cox MM. Lehninger Principles of Biochemistry. Macmillan; 2008.

8. Berg JM, Tymoczko JL, Stryer L et al. Biochemistry & Bioportal. W H Freeman & Company; 2011.

9. Garrett R, Grisham C. Biochemistry. Cengage Learning; 2012.

10. Satyanarayana U. Biochemistry. 2006.

11. Robert H. Herman, David Zakim. Fructose Metabolism. The American Journal of Clinical Nutrition Vol. 21, No. 3, March 1968. pp. 245-249.

12. Goldberg T, Slonim AE. Nutrition therapy for hepatic glycogen storage diseases. J Am Diet Assoc. 1993;93(12):1423-30.

13. Paschos P, Paletas K. Non alcoholic fatty liver disease and metabolic syndrome. Hippokratia. 2009;13(1):9-19.

14. Chedid A, Mendenhall CL, Gartside P, French SW, Chen T, Rabin L. Prognostic factors in alcoholic liver disease. VA Cooperative Study Group. Am J Gastroenterol. 1991;86(2):210-6.

15. National Diabetes Information Clearinghouse. Hypoglycemia. Web. 17 March 2015.

16. Yoneyama S, Sakurai M, Nakamura K, et al. Associations between rice, noodle, and bread intake and sleep quality in Japanese men and women. PLoS ONE. 2014;9(8):e105198.

17. Lee BM, Wolever TM. Effect of glucose, sucrose and fructose on plasma glucose and insulin responses in normal humans: comparison with white bread. Eur J Clin Nutr. 1998;52(12):924-8.

18. Atkinson FS, Foster-powell K, Brand-miller JC. International tables of glycemic index and glycemic load values: 2008. Diabetes Care. 2008;31(12):2281-3.

19. Shambaugh P, Worthington V, Herbert JH. Differential effects of honey, sucrose, and fructose on blood sugar levels. J Manipulative Physiol Ther. 1990;13(6):322-5.

20. Cozma AI, Sievenpiper JL, De souza RJ, et al. Effect of fructose on glycemic control in diabetes: a systematic review and meta-analysis of controlled feeding trials. Diabetes Care. 2012;35(7):1611-20.

21. Heacock PM, Hertzler SR, Wolf BW. Fructose prefeeding reduces the glycemic response to a high-glycemic index, starchy food in humans. J Nutr. 2002;132(9):2601-4.

22. Sautin YY, Johnson RJ. Uric acid: the oxidant-antioxidant paradox. Nucleosides Nucleotides Nucleic Acids. 2008;27(6):608-19.

23. Ames BN, Cathcart R, Schwiers E, Hochstein P. Uric acid provides an antioxidant defense in humans against oxidant – and radical-caused aging and cancer: a hypothesis. Proc Natl Acad Sci USA. 1981;78(11):6858-62.

24. Gutman AB, Yu TF. Renal regulation of uric acid excretion in normal and gouty man; modification by uricosuric agents. Bull N Y Acad Med. 1958;34(5):287-96.

25. Schatz IJ, Masaki K, Yano K, Chen R, Rodriguez BL, Curb JD. Cholesterol and all-cause mortality in elderly people from the Honolulu Heart Program: a cohort study. Lancet. 2001 Aug 4;358(9279):351-5.

26. Smith LL. Another cholesterol hypothesis: cholesterol as antioxidant. Free Radic Biol Med. 1991;11(1):47-61.

27. Payne AH, Hales DB. Overview of steroidogenic enzymes in the pathway from cholesterol to active steroid hormones. Endocr Rev. 2004;25(6):947-70.

28. H. Vierhapper H, Nardi A, Grösser P, Raber W, Gessl A. Low-density lipoprotein cholesterol in subclinical hypothyroidism. Thyroid. 2000;10(11):981-4.

29. Cachefo A, Boucher P, Vidon C, Dusserre E, Diraison F, Beylot M. Hepatic lipogenesis and cholesterol synthesis in hyperthyroid patients. J Clin Endocrinol Metab. 2001;86(11):5353-7.

30. White LW, Landau BR. SUGAR TRANSPORT AND FRUCTOSE METABOLISM IN HUMAN INTESTINE IN VITRO. J Clin Invest. 1965;44:1200-13.

31. White JS. Straight talk about high-fructose corn syrup: what it is and what it ain't. Am J Clin Nutr. 2008;88(6):1716S-1721S.

32. Lecoultre V, Benoit R, Carrel G, et al. Fructose and glucose co-ingestion during prolonged exercise increases lactate and glucose fluxes and oxidation compared with an equimolar intake of glucose. Am J Clin Nutr. 2010;92(5):1071-9.

33. Yasutake K, Kohjima M, Kotoh K, Nakashima M, Nakamuta M, Enjoji M. Dietary habits and behaviors associated with nonalcoholic fatty liver disease. World J Gastroenterol. 2014;20(7):1756-67.

34. Leevy CM. Fatty liver: a study of 270 patients with biopsy proven fatty liver and review of the literature. Medicine (Baltimore). 1962;41:249-76.

35. Corbin KD, Zeisel SH. Choline metabolism provides novel insights into nonalcoholic fatty liver disease and its progression. Curr Opin Gastroenterol. 2012;28(2):159-65.

36. Buchman AL, Ament ME, Sohel M, et al. Choline deficiency causes reversible hepatic abnormalities in patients receiving parenteral nutrition: proof of a human choline requirement: a placebo-controlled trial. JPEN J Parenter Enteral Nutr. 2001;25(5):260-8.

Chapter 6: Let's Look at Honey

1. Gheldof N, Wang XH, Engeseth NJ. Identification and quantification of antioxidant components of honeys from various floral sources. J Agric Food Chem. 2002;50:5870–7.

2. Bogdanov S, Jurendic T, Sieber R. et al. Honey for nutrition and health: a review. J Am Coll Nutr.2008;27:677–89.

3. Jan Mei, S., 2 Mohd Nordin, M. S. and 3,*Norrakiah, A. S. Fructooligosaccharides in honey and effects of honey on growth of Bifidobacterium longum BB 536. International Food Research Journal 17: 557-561 (2010)

4. Michele R. Warmund. Department of Horticulture, University of Missouri. Pollinating Fruit Crops. http://extension.missouri.edu/p/g6001

5. Rajan TV, Tennen H, Lindquist RL, Cohen L, Clive J. Effect of ingestion of honey on symptoms of rhinoconjunctivitis. Ann Allergy Asthma Immunol. 2002 Feb;88(2):198-203.

6. Bogdanov S. Contaminants of bee products. Apidologie. 2006;38:1–18.

7. Schneider A. Asian honey, banned in Europe, is flooding U.S. grocery shelves. 7. The Food Watchdog, Seattle Washington; 2011. Assessed from http://www.foodsafetynews.com/2011/08/honey-laundering/ on 14/04/12.

8. Frankel SM, Robbinson GE, Berenbaum MR. Antioxidant capacity and correlated characteristics of 14 unifloral honeys. J Apicultural Res. 1998;37:27–31

9. Earnest CP, Lancaster SL, Rasmussen CJ, et al. Low vs. high glycemic index carbohydrate gel ingestion during simulated 64-km cycling time trial performance. J Strength Cond Res. 2004;18(3):466-72.

10. Heman RH, Zakim D. Fructose metabolism. I. The fructose metabolic pathway. Am J Clin Nutr. 1968 Mar; 21(3):245-9.

11. Schramm DD, Karim M, Schrader HR, Holt RR, Cardetti M, Keen CL. Honey with high levels of antioxidants can provide protection to healthy human subjects. J Agric Food Chem. 2003;51(6):1732-5.

12. Al-waili NS, Haq A. Effect of honey on antibody production against thymus-dependent and thymus-independent antigens in primary and secondary immune responses. J Med Food. 2004;7(4):491-4.

13. Molan PC. The potential of honey to promote oral wellness. Gen Dent. 2001;49(6):584-9.

14. English HK, Pack AR, Molan PC. The effects of manuka honey on plaque and gingivitis: a pilot study. J Int Acad Periodontol. 2004;6(2):63-7.

15. Grobler SR, Du toit IJ, Basson NJ. The effect of honey on human tooth enamel in vitro observed by electron microscopy and microhardness measurements. Arch Oral Biol. 1994;39(2):147-53.

16. Ali ATMM. Natural honey accelerates healing of indomethacin induced antral ulcers in rats. Saudi Med J. 1995;16:161–166

17. Molan P. Why honey is effective as a medicine. 2. The scientific explanation of its effects. Bee World. 2001;82:22–40.

18. Emarah MH. A clinical study of the topical use of bee honey in the treatment of some occular diseases. Bull Islam Med.1982;2(5):422–425.

19. Al-waili NS. Natural honey lowers plasma glucose, C-reactive protein, homocysteine, and blood lipids in healthy, diabetic, and hyperlipidemic subjects: comparison with dextrose and sucrose. J Med Food. 2004;7(1):100-7.

20. Al-Waili NS, Saloom KY. Effects of topical honey on post-operative wound infections due to gram positive and gram negative bacteria following caesarean sections and hysterectomies. Eur J Med Res. 1999 Mar 26; 4(3):126-30.

21. Erejuwa OO, Sulaiman SA, Wahab MS. Review Oligosaccharides might contribute to the antidiabetic effect of honey: a review of the literature. Molecules. 2011 Dec 28; 17(1):248-66.

22. Conlee RK, Lawler RM, Ross PE. Effects of glucose or fructose feeding on glycogen repletion in muscle and liver after exercise or fasting. Ann Nutr Metab. 1987;31(2):126-32.

23. Visser TJ, Kaptein E, Terpstra OT, Krenning EP. Deiodination of thyroid hormone by human liver. J Clin Endocrinol Metab. 1988 Jul;67(1):17-24.

24. De Pedro N, Delgado MJ, Gancedo B, Alonso-Bedate M. Changes in glucose, glycogen, thyroid activity and hypothalamic catecholamines in tench by starvation and refeeding. J Comp Physiol B. 2003 Aug;173(6):475-81. Epub 2003 May 21.

25. Stephen W. Spaulding, Inder J. Chopra, Robert S. Sherwin and Santokh S. Lyall. EFFECT OF CALORIC RESTRICTION AND DIETARY COMPOSITION ON SERUM T3 AND REVERSE T3 IN MAN. The Journal of Clinical Endocrinology & Metabolism January 1, 1976 vol. 42 no. 1 197-200

26. Abrams JJ, Grundy SM. Cholesterol metabolism in hypothyroidism and hyperthyroidism in man. J Lipid Res. 1981 Feb;22(2):323-38.

27. Elder J, McLelland A, O'Reilly DS, Packard CJ, Series JJ, Shepherd J. The relationship between serum cholesterol and serum thyrotropin, thyroxine and tri-iodothyronine concentrations in suspected hypothyroidism. Ann Clin Biochem. 1990 Mar;27 (Pt 2):110-3.

28. Teff KL, Elliott SS, Tschöp M, et al. Dietary fructose reduces circulating insulin and leptin, attenuates postprandial suppression of ghrelin, and increases triglycerides in women. J Clin Endocrinol Metab. 2004;89(6):2963-72.

29. Erejuwa OO, Sulaiman SA, Wahab MS. Fructose might contribute to the hypoglycemic effect of honey. Molecules. 2012;17:1900–15.

Chapter 7: What about Diabetes 2?

1. Engelgau MM, Thompson TJ, Herman WH, et al. Comparison of fasting and 2-hour glucose and HbA1c levels for diagnosing diabetes. Diagnostic criteria and performance revisited. Diabetes Care. 1997;20(5):785-91.

2. Crawford SO, Hoogeveen RC, Brancati FL, et al. Association of blood lactate with type 2 diabetes: the Atherosclerosis Risk in Communities Carotid MRI Study. Int J Epidemiol. 2010;39(6):1647-55.

3. Bugianesi E, Moscatiello S, Ciaravella MF, Marchesini G. Insulin resistance in nonalcoholic fatty liver disease. Curr Pharm Des. 2010;16(17):1941-51.

4. Wong VW, Wong GL, Yeung DK, et al. Fatty pancreas, insulin resistance, and β-cell function: a population study using fat-water magnetic resonance imaging. Am J Gastroenterol. 2014;109(4):589-97.

5. Bryan RN, Bilello M, Davatzikos C, et al. Effect of diabetes on brain structure: the action to control cardiovascular risk in diabetes MR imaging baseline data. Radiology. 2014;272(1):210-6.

6. De la monte SM, Wands JR. Alzheimer's disease is type 3 diabetes-evidence reviewed. J Diabetes Sci Technol. 2008;2(6):1101-13.

Chapter 8: The Fat Chapter

1. Summers LK, Barnes SC, Fielding BA, et al. Uptake of individual fatty acids into adipose tissue in relation to their presence in the diet. Am J Clin Nutr. 2000;71(6):1470-7.

2. Field CJ, Angel A, Clandinin MT. Relationship of diet to the fatty acid composition of human adipose tissue structural and stored lipids. Am J Clin Nutr. 1985;42(6):1206-20.

3. Jo J, Gavrilova O, Pack S, et al. Hypertrophy and/or Hyperplasia: Dynamics of Adipose Tissue Growth. PLoS Comput Biol. 2009;5(3):e1000324.

4. Lanier JS, Corl BA. Challenges in enriching milk fat with polyunsaturated fatty acids. J Anim Sci Biotechnol. 2015;6(1):26.

5. Rahman K. Studies on free radicals, antioxidants, and co-factors. Clin Interv Aging. 2007;2(2):219-36.

6. Leyton J, Drury PJ, Crawford MA. Differential oxidation of saturated and unsaturated fatty acids in vivo in the rat. Br J Nutr. 1987;57(3):383-93.

7. Michal Bachar,Patrick Brunelle,D. Peter Tieleman, Arvi Rauk*. Molecular Dynamics Simulation of a Polyunsaturated Lipid Bilayer Susceptible to Lipid Peroxidation. The Journal of Physical Chemistry B 2004 108 (22), 7170-7179.

8. Schrauwen P, Hesselink MK. Oxidative capacity, lipotoxicity, and mitochondrial damage in type 2 diabetes. Diabetes. 2004;53(6):1412-7.

Chapter 9: Protein

1. Magnusson I, Rothman DL, Katz LD, Shulman RG, Shulman GI. Increased rate of gluconeogenesis in type II diabetes mellitus. A 13C nuclear magnetic resonance study. J Clin Invest. 1992;90(4):1323-7.

2. Yin M, Ikejima K, Arteel GE, et al. Glycine accelerates recovery from alcohol-induced liver injury. J Pharmacol Exp Ther. 1998;286(2):1014-9.

3. Sidransky H. Role of tryptophan in carcinogenesis. Adv Exp Med Biol. 1986;206:187-207.

4. Carvalho DP, Ferreira AC, Coelho SM, Moraes JM, Camacho MA, Rosenthal D. Thyroid peroxidase activity is inhibited by amino acids. Braz J Med Biol Res. 2000;33(3):355-61.

5. Mezey E. Liver disease and protein needs. Annu Rev Nutr. 1982;2:21-50.

Chapter 10: Stress

1. Chandola T, Brunner E, Marmot M. Chronic stress at work and the metabolic syndrome: prospective study. BMJ. 2006;332(7540):521-5.

2. Kiecolt-glaser JK, Preacher KJ, Maccallum RC, Atkinson C, Malarkey WB, Glaser R. Chronic stress and age-related increases in the proinflammatory cytokine IL-6. Proc Natl Acad Sci USA. 2003;100(15):9090-5.

3. Schiffrin, Holly and S., Nelson, (2010), Stressed and Happy? Investigating the Relationship Between Happiness and Perceived Stress, Journal of Happiness Studies, 11, issue 1, p. 33-39.

4. Berlett BS, Stadtman ER. Protein oxidation in aging, disease, and oxidative stress. J Biol Chem. 1997;272(33):20313-6.

5. Defining and reporting hypoglycemia in diabetes: a report from the American Diabetes Association Workgroup on Hypoglycemia. Diabetes Care. 2005;28(5):1245-9.

Chapter 11: Vitamins and Minerals

1. Heaney RP, Weaver CM, Recker RR. Calcium absorbability from spinach. Am J Clin Nutr. 1988;47(4):707-9.

Chapter 12: The First Diet Revealed

1. Weinberg, Bennett Alan; Bealer, Bonnie K (2001). The World of Caffeine: The Science and Culture of the World's Most Popular Drug. pp. 3–4.

2. Acheson KJ, Zahorska-markiewicz B, Pittet P, Anantharaman K, Jéquier E. Caffeine and coffee: their influence on metabolic rate and substrate utilization in normal weight and obese individuals. Am J Clin Nutr. 1980;33(5):989-97.

3. Nakanishi N, Nakamura K, Suzuki K, Tatara K. Effects of coffee consumption against the development of liver dysfunction: a 4-year follow-up study of middle-aged Japanese male office workers. Ind Health. 2000;38(1):99-102.

4. Kono S, Shinchi K, Imanishi K, Todoroki I, Hatsuse K. Coffee and serum gamma-glutamyltransferase: a study of self-defense officials in Japan. Am J Epidemiol. 1994;139(7):723-7.

5. Ross GW, Abbott RD, Petrovitch H, et al. Association of coffee and caffeine intake with the risk of Parkinson disease. JAMA. 2000;283(20):2674-9.

6. Van dam RM, Willett WC, Manson JE, Hu FB. Coffee, caffeine, and risk of type 2 diabetes: a prospective cohort study in younger and middle-aged U.S. women. Diabetes Care. 2006;29(2):398-403.

7. Crozier SJ, Preston AG, Hurst JW, et al. Cacao seeds are a "Super Fruit": A comparative analysis of various fruit powders and products. Chem Cent J. 2011;5(1):5.

8. Sorond FA, Hurwitz S, Salat DH, Greve DN, Fisher ND. Neurovascular coupling, cerebral white matter integrity, and response to cocoa in older people. Neurology. 2013;81(10):904-9.

9. Cuenca-garcía M, Ruiz JR, Ortega FB, Castillo MJ. Association between chocolate consumption and fatness in European adolescents. Nutrition. 2014;30(2):236-9.

10. J. Kubola, S. Siriamornpun and N. Meeso, "Phytochemicals, Vitamin C and Sugar Content of Thai Wild Fruits," Food Chemistry, Vol. 126, No. 3, 2011, pp. 972-981.

11. Cooperation DS, Affairs PA, Council NR. Lost Crops of Africa:, Volume II: Vegetables. National Academies Press; 2006.

12. JR Minkel. Earliest Known Seafood Dinner Discovered. Scientific American. Oct 17, 2007.

13. "TUKUL 1: African Prehistory". Sapienza Universita Di Roma. Web. September 9th 2015.
http://www.melkakunture.it/museum/tukul1-06.html

Chapter 15: Carbohydrates, Protein, and Fat

1. Nagy TR, Goran MI, Weinsier RL, Toth MJ, Schutz Y, Poehlman ET. Determinants of basal fat oxidation in healthy Caucasians. J Appl Physiol. 1996;80(5):1743-8.

Chapter 18: The First Diet Workouts

1. Nikolaidis MG, Kyparos A, Spanou C, Paschalis V, Theodorou AA, Vrabas IS. Redox biology of exercise: an integrative and comparative consideration of some overlooked issues. J Exp Biol. 2012;215(Pt 10):1615-25.

Chapter 20: One Last Word on the Limitations of Diet

1. Chinnery PF. Muscle Diseases. In: Goldman L, Schafer AI, eds. Goldman's Cecil Medicine. 24th ed. Philadelphia, PA: Saunders Elsevier; 2011:chap 429.

31859850R10141

Made in the USA
San Bernardino, CA
21 March 2016